MW01257683

Patrick Bouvier Kennedy

Michael S. Ryan, RRT-NPS

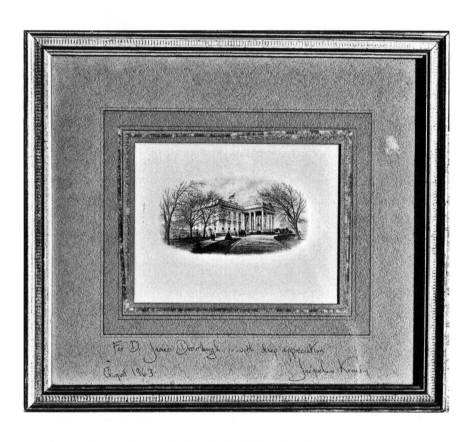

Received as a gift from Jackie Kennedy, a framed portrait
of the White House signed by the First Lady thanking Dr.
James Drorbaugh for his efforts to help save Patrick.
(August 1963)
(Photograph by James E. Drorbaugh Jr., Kaneohe, Hawaii)

Patrick Bouvier Kennedy

A Brief Life That Changed the History of Newborn Care

Michael S. Ryan, RRT-NPS

MCP BOOKS, MINNEAPOLIS

Copyright © 2015 by Michael S. Ryan, RRT - NPS

MCP Books
322 First Avenue N, 5th floor
Minneapolis, MN 55401
612.455.2293

All rights reserved. No part of this publication may be reproduced,
stored in a retrieval system, or transmitted, in any form or by
any means, electronic, mechanical, photocopying, recording, or
otherwise, without the prior written permission of the author.

ISBN-13: 978-1-63413-590-0
LCCN: 2015908940

Distributed by Itasca Books

Cover Design by Andre Bat
Typeset by Colleen Rollins

Printed in the United States of America

To Judy,
my parents Leo (Sonny) and Julia Ryan,
and the Babies

From the child of five to myself is but a step. But from the newborn baby to the child of five is an appalling distance.
—Leo Tolstoi (1828–1910)

Contents

Acknowledgments.. *viii*

Introduction .... *xii*

1. A Time to Be Born 1

2. The Tears of a Mother 3

3. The Historical Baby... 6

4. Coming of Age: The Preterm Baby 14

5. The Sanitarians... 18

6. Naming Respiratory Distress Syndrome 24

7. Patrick's Birth.. 40

8. The First Breath... 47

9. The Infant Lung... 50

10. Patrick's Desperate Hours 60

11. Prayers for a Baby.. 63

12. Patrick's Death 71

13. Hope for the Newborn at Risk 83

14. May Children Have Light 93

15. Behind-the-Scenes Interviews: The Three Days That
   Changed Everything.. 96
   James Drorbaugh, MD, James Hughes, MD,
   and William Bernhard, MD

Bibliography... 131

Acknowledgments

My deepest gratitude goes to James Drorbaugh, MD, William Bernhard, MD, and James Hughes, MD, who freely discussed with me their highly personal associations with Patrick Bouvier Kennedy, the details of which, before this volume, had never been spoken of publicly. The three physicians were at the center of the Patrick Bouvier Kennedy medical crisis as it unfolded. Their generous allotment of time for personal meetings, phone calls, and tape-recorded conversations has resulted in interviews printed in the rear of this book. Offering many unique details surrounding the life and death of Patrick Bouvier Kennedy, their substantial contributions to this book are immeasurable and my debt to them incalculable.

I have also benefited from the help and encouragement of other people. A special acknowledgment goes to Nicholas M. Nelson, MD (1922–2014), whose death I mourned during the final stages of this book. I met "Nick," a pioneer in neonatal physiology, halfway through the writing of this book. His critique of earlier drafts and enthusiastic encouragement combined to help propel the project forward. He was a beacon in the discipline of neonatal respiratory care, and I hope the final version of this book would have elicited Dr. Nelson's approval.

My deepest admiration also goes to Will Cochran, MD, a pediatrician at the Boston Lying-in Hospital (now the Brigham and Women's Hospital). Although Dr. Cochran happened to be on vacation when the Kennedy baby arrived, his generous input and anecdotal reflections on the care of preterm babies in the late 1950s and early 1960s were invaluable in allowing me to set the tone of the early Boston special care nursery.

Special thanks also to Dr. Welton Gersony, former Alexander S.

Nadas Professor of Pediatric Cardiology at Columbia University and director of pediatric cardiology at Morgan Stanley Children's Hospital. As a pediatric cardiology fellow in 1963, Dr. Gersony's eyewitness account of those gathered around the president's baby embodies the kind of moment in which a writer takes great joy.

I am also deeply indebted to Avery Fanaroff, MD, a Virginia Apgar awardee, coeditor of *Care of the High Risk Neonate,* and coauthor of Fanaroff and Martin's *Neonatal–Perinatal Medicine,* who kindly took the time to express his view on the impact of Patrick's untimely death on modern neonatal care.

I would also like to thank everyone who read all or part of my manuscript: Bob Baker, Lin Thompson, RN, Kimberly Cheng, RN, David Cheng, MD, Michael Indgin, Michael Lash, Carolyn Ward, Keith Kolber, MD, Michelle Henry, MD, Glenda Minjares, RN, and Mace and Carolyn Perlman. A special thanks also to Laurie Kney, for her graphic design work.

Also a very special thanks to Elizabeth Kaye, whose editorial eye for clarity and content helped me to shape this book. Her encouragement to stay the narrative course, while avoiding lengthy expositions, added immensely to the quality of the manuscript.

My tremendous appreciation also goes to Holly Montieth, my extraordinary editor, who not only regularly reassured me when I became uncertain but whose expert eye for detail and flow helped guide the book to its final presentation.

I also wish to acknowledge the numerous medical historians, scientists, and academics whose books and papers offered me the historical commentary necessary to support my research, all of whom are cited or listed in the rear of the book.

Finally, thanks to my wife, Judy McLaughlin-Ryan, for her patience and unflagging support during the writing of this book, as throughout our entire marriage. Judy was also my first draft reader and the first to point out my narratives gone astray. Her simple acts of keeping my health and well-being balanced throughout the writing of this book revealed a steadfast dedication to the vows of Holy Matrimony that we undertook some twenty-odd years ago. On the day we met, as now, there remains something deeply touching and appealing in her nature, and it is with honor and humility that I subject her to a similar loyalty affirming my marital promise "until death do us part."

Introduction

In the summer of 1989 at three o'clock in the morning, I was standing inside a neonatal intensive care unit watching a baby nearing death. I was then, as now, working as a registered respiratory therapist specializing in newborn care; the baby, whom I will call Christy, was born at thirty-four weeks' gestation and weighed four and a half pounds, or 2,050 grams. She was only three hours old and breathing at a rate well past a hundred breaths a minute. Despite being on a ventilator and receiving 100 percent oxygen, the little girl's skin color was pale and blue. I held in my hand a small vial of fluid containing a milk-like substance that carried the trademark name of Survanta and was, at that time, a new drug. Created from minced bovine (cow) lung containing pulmonary surfactant used to treat infant respiratory distress syndrome, it had been in the making for more than twenty years. I squirted it directly into a breathing tube leading into Christy's lungs.

Within seconds, the baby's skin color went from blue to pink, and her breathing rate quickly descended into a more normal range. Standing at the head of the bed with me that morning was an attending neonatologist. We marveled at the rapidity of the drug's effect, at the way it had changed this mortally ill infant into a newborn flush full of life and health—and had done so within seconds.

Standing shoulder to shoulder with this veteran doctor, I could tell that he was as thrilled as I was by the baby's remarkable turnaround.

The doctor then remarked, "The Kennedy baby died at thirty-four weeks' gestation, and look at this now!"

I replied, "The Kennedy baby? Who's that?"

"He was the president's baby boy who died from respiratory distress syndrome. He's the one who started it all."

Looking back now, the doctor's offhand remark about "the one who started it all" summarizes Patrick Bouvier Kennedy's contribution to newborn care research and would, twenty years later, lead me to write this book. Despite the fact that, for decades, researchers worldwide focusing on respiratory care of the premature infant would often cite respiratory distress syndrome as the disease that killed the president's son, more than fifty years since Patrick's death, no one has told the entire and dramatic tale of Patrick's doomed struggle for life, of his parents' consummate grace and courage in the face of tragedy, and of how his death came to impact modern newborn care.

Blessed with the enormous good fortune to acquire the very first, full-length interviews with physicians directly involved in Patrick's care, I use their firsthand testimony to add immensely to the riveting story of the event that "started it all."

How It All Started

On August 7, 1963, Patrick Bouvier Kennedy was born the second son of President and Mrs. John F. Kennedy. The birth of the baby to an enormously popular presidential couple created an immediate national celebration, and its effect was felt worldwide. Three days later, it was announced to a startled public that Patrick, at thirty-four weeks' gestational age, had died from a common lung ailment known as hyaline membrane disease (HMD), now called respiratory distress syndrome (RDS).

The heavily publicized event provoked a strong worldwide political and social reaction. News of Patrick's death took precedence in all major American and European newspapers, prompting personal letters of condolence from countless heads of state and religious leaders, including Pope Paul VI. The Soviet news agency Tass, then an instrument for the promotion of anti-Western bias, compassionately included the tragic news in its daily broadcast. The White House sent out more than thirty-five thousand acknowledgments in response to cards received from people unknown to the Kennedys, expressing condolences over the lost infant.

Capturing the emotions of a public that loved its president and first lady, Patrick's death was soon lost to public memory only a few months later by his father's death in Dallas. However, the stage had been set. Patrick's death focused national attention on the malady that killed him, RDS, which, at the time, claimed the lives of twenty--five thousand babies a year in the United States alone. The scientific investigations that would follow the little boy's brief life would spark a revolution in newborn medical research, resulting in the saving of thousands of babies per year, a legacy that continues.

The Legacy of a Brief Life

What began as a book about the Kennedy baby's life would, by necessity, expand into the much larger field of newborn history. By including beginning chapters devoted to a history of newborn care, placing emphasis on the West, in particular, on America, my intent is to acquaint the reader with the larger social context in which the crucial moments of Patrick's life took place. The historical overview, however brief, suffices to help the reader gain perspective on how the prevention of infant deaths by RDS is a relatively new concept in clinical medicine.

Patrick's death in 1963 brought focus to a process of development that began in 1903 with the discovery of a lung ailment that was fatal for infants. Starting as a series of discoveries known only to a few scientists working within the narrow field of newborn lung disease, there was little physicians could do to intervene in the lung disease process. The government did not take the problem seriously, and the public was unaware of how many babies died as a result of RDS until Patrick's death in 1963.

RDS, in claiming its most prominent victim while drawing public focus onto the lung ailment, would also invigorate scientific investigation into its cause. The consequences of those actions would lead the National Institute of Child Health and Development (NICHD) to announce, in 2012, in a listing of long-range mission and scientific accomplishments, that "since becoming operative in 1963 under the Kennedy administration, the NICHD highlights as its number one accomplishment [that] the survival rates for Respiratory Distress Syndrome have gone from 5% in the 1960s, to 95% today."[1]

Because Patrick lived and died, many infants born today with RDS are no longer living under a death sentence. Today, countless infants who suffered from RDS have been spared and gone on to lead healthy lives as a direct result of Patrick's tragically brief but significant existence.

Overview

Although I was assisted by many special individuals, the writing of this book was foremost a solitary pursuit, an undertaking that spread itself over a long period of time. During this time, my keen interest in the project was augmented by my continuing work as a newborn intensive care unit (NICU) respiratory care practitioner based in a Los Angeles inner-city hospital. My goal in writing the book was to help clarify the link between Patrick Bouvier Kennedy's death and its impact on newborn lung research and how these studies would advance respiratory care of the newborn, leading to improved survival of the preterm baby.

In my attempt to address the book to a general audience, I paid careful attention not to inundate the reader with technical details. For the historian and those familiar with clinical newborn care, there are areas of the book where extrapolations of scientific and historical detail were avoided both to help the flow of the story and to minimize the inevitable misunderstandings such details would arouse in the general reader. Beginning with chapter 6 and continuing to the end of the book, much of my source material is taken directly from interviews I conducted, which are printed in the back of the book.

Because the history of newborn care touches so much human activity over such a large span of time, no single book could include everything and everyone, and so this book is not intended to be a complete treatise on the subject. For this reason, I apologize for any persons or aspects of newborn history that I may have omitted; for those wishing to investigate on their own, a bibliography of resource material is included.

1. http://www.nichd.nih.gov/about/overview/mission/Pages/index.aspx

The death of Patrick Bouvier Kennedy was a seminal event in the history of neonatal care. His death spurred the creation of what is now the Shriver National Institute of Child Health and Human Development, which accelerated research that has been translated from the bench to the bedside. Within a decade of his death, there was a much better understanding of respiratory distress syndrome, resulting in a more rational approach to therapy and better outcomes. The development of ventilators specifically designed for neonates and the introduction of CPAP [continuous positive airway pressure] dramatically improved survival rates, which increased even more with the introduction of surfactant therapy some twenty years later. Today, babies with a similar birth weight and gestational age to Patrick Kennedy would have a 99 percent chance of survival.[2]

---

2. Dr. Avroy Fanaroff, author and Virginia Apgar Award recipient, personal communication with the author, 2014.

1

A Time to Be Born

Every time a child is born it brings with it the hope
that God is not yet disappointed with man.
—Rabrindranath Tagore (1861–1941)

As a respiratory care practitioner and twenty-five-year veteran of the
neonatal intensive care unit at my hospital, I have attended the deliveries of well over ten thousand high-risk infants, many of whom were premature. Nowadays, happily, the overwhelming majority of premature
infants are routinely treated and discharged, without fanfare, from hospital to home and soon become indistinguishable in physiology from
their born-at-term counterparts.

Yet, despite tremendous advances in infant care made over recent
decades, there remain those special infants born with biological limitations: congenital liabilities or various biological aberrations. For these
infants, cardiopulmonary homeostasis is quickly pushed to its limit, at
which point the process of dying ensues.

I have had what I consider to be the holy privilege to have been
involved in the care of countless such infants—God's babies, as some
would call them—while they are dying and at the moment of their
deaths.

For those in my profession, observing an infant or child die is not an exercise in clinical detachment. To watch a baby die is to be consumed by two deeply troubling and confusing thoughts: the first is our powerlessness in the face of death; the second is how brutal nature can be.

Each of these sensations prompts feelings of helplessness, leading sadly and inevitably to the knowledge that there is not a damn thing you can do about either.

To see an innocent newborn die produces such tidal waves of emotion that these deaths are rarely discussed among clinicians involved in clinical newborn and pediatric care, who may perhaps experience a mysterious spiritual connection with the infants for whom they care. This connection may occur at a level that bypasses ordinary thought and feeling, so much so that the caretaker is often unaware of its existence until he or she is in the middle of some routine household chore and suddenly begins to weep uncontrollably for a baby who has died. Much to the bewilderment of others, these unbidden feelings can suddenly erupt while a person is taking out the trash or watching a TV comedy or a sunset.

Of the babies whose deaths I have personally witnessed, many were born extremely premature and afflicted with associated RDS. When President Kennedy and his wife, Jacqueline, lost Patrick just thirty-nine hours after birth, they joined thousands of parents of the era whose children had died soon after birth because of RDS. Parents, then as now, almost always perceive the loss of a child as a senseless act of God.

Following Patrick's death, the president mourned deeply, but his unique position would ultimately turn his bereavement into political legislation that would transform newborn infant care. Because of the president's loss, many babies and parents no longer suffer the ravages of RDS.

2

The Tears of a Mother

Unto the woman he said, I will greatly multiply thy sorrow and
thy conception; in sorrow though shalt bring forth children.
—Genesis 3:16, King James Version

Effective newborn care is a recent development that evolved at the expense of an enormous human sacrifice. In the United States, as late as the early 1960s, countless parents were subjected to the loss of a newborn, a tragedy that can leave many psychologically and spiritually scarred for life.

I recently visited one such parent who lost a baby in 1960. Now, she is eighty-two years old, a small, white-haired woman with a simple spirit, an open heart, and memories that remain painful and vivid.

Her second-born son, named Leonard, died as a result of, as she puts it, "the same thing that killed the Kennedy kid." She is referring to RDS, which was known at the time as hyaline membrane disease and which she calls "Haley Member's" disease. Her mispronunciation strikes me as sweet and prompts a smile that disappears the moment she begins to recount her story.

Leonard was born premature at thirty-two weeks' gestation. "He looked big and healthy," she recalls, and he was crying like mad. . . . I saw him for only a couple of minutes, and then he was taken away. The next day my doctor came into my room and told me in a matter-of-fact way that Lenny was dead. He didn't tell me much more than that, only saying Lenny began to have a hard time breathing after he was born. He also mentioned I was young and my uterus was in good shape so I shouldn't have any problems having another baby. He seemed to be in a hurry when he gave me the news and didn't even tell me good-bye. When he left my room, I started crying and couldn't stop. I kept hearing Lenny cry even though he was dead and this [the sound of Lenny crying] lasted for a couple days. To make matters worse, Bob [her husband] took it hard and began to drink heavily, which made him really mean to me. Before I knew it, I had a nervous breakdown and had to spend another two weeks in the hospital. I felt like a huge failure as a woman and a wife and felt so sick and ashamed of Lenny's death, thinking somehow it was my fault. I never told anyone about it until the little Kennedy boy died. That's when I found out the Haley's disease killed a lot of babies. I guess it made me feel better knowing it just wasn't me.

As it turns out, she was far from the only parent who kept her child's death a secret until the death of Patrick Bouvier Kennedy. In a sense, this isn't surprising: in the 1960s, John and Jackie Kennedy were models for myriad things—from having what JFK in his Bostonian accent called "vigah" (vigor) to Jackie's pillbox hats. The knowledge that RDS had devastated America's most glamorous and powerful pair allowed scores of parents to feel they had been granted permission to openly discuss a newborn's death rather than feeling consigned to treating it as something dark, shameful, and unspeakable.

After Patrick's death, public health officials began to weigh in on the matter of RDS. Medical scientists worldwide began to explore this puzzling respiratory disease that Patrick's death had catapulted into a medical issue of national importance.

America, an affluent nation unlike any other, was uniquely

positioned to devote scientific talent and economic resources to finding a cure for the disease that, in the 1960s, killed twenty-five thousand infants in the United States each year, among them the second son of Jack and Jackie Kennedy.

3

The Historical Baby

Here pretty baby lye's
Sung asleep with lullabies
Pray be silent and not stir
The earth that covers her.
　　　　—early gravestone epitaph, unknown author

Infants form a unique society and, in a sense, a special nation of their own. The terms we employ when referring to them—"small wonders," "little miracles," and "nature's blessings"—suggest that human newborns belong to realms of both nature and spirit. The newborn readily instills parental devotion and can open the most steeled of hearts; it can alter the human psyche and transform even the most self-centered and self-serving individuals into people capable of sacrifice, caring, and love for other human beings.

Because of my long NICU experience, I also view the infant as the original diplomatic envoy of the human spirit and as the bedrock of civilized humanity. The exalted nature of infants is one of the many reasons the World Health Organization in 1950 wisely adopted the infant mortality rate as an index of national health.[3]

---

3. The *infant mortality rate* is defined as the number of infant deaths occurring at one year of age or younger per one thousand live births.

To understand how far we have come, and how far we still need to go, a brief, historical review of newborn care is in order. The account will give the reader perspective on the evolution of newborn medicine, in particular innovations that occurred leading up to the death of Patrick Bouvier Kennedy and those that followed.

Early Western Beginnings

In the long-distant view of our Greek medical heritage dating back to 460 B.C., it is noteworthy that the prevention of newborn death is a relatively new concept in human history. History tells us that more than two thousand years had elapsed before any serious efforts were put into marking the medical beginnings of the newborn care tradition, most of which did not begin until the twentieth century. Furthermore, a review of newborn care stretching back to ancient times reveals a near-total absence of systematized infant medical knowledge—a mystery in its own right. In the minds of our primitive ancestors, human infant care was inseparable from religious belief, relegating the newborn throughout millennia to a place subordinate to nature, myth, and superstition.[4] During this early period in Europe, treatises discussing infant and childhood disease were rarely written. These studies, few in number, were like tiny flickers of light cast against the much brighter and broader landscape of adult medical investigation. It was not until the middle part of the twentieth century that serious scientific investigations into infant and child care would accelerate.

A further look into the long, narrow course of newborn history reveals a deeper and darker truth: that the practices of child abandonment and infanticide were socially accepted solutions to disposing of unwanted babies and children. This was the case despite the fact that, culturally, much was made of the sacred connection between mother and child. Consider, for instance, the glorious religious art of the Italian

---

4. In actuality, we have little information about the daily lives of infants in the medieval world. "Our ancestors left few records bearing on the subject [infancy]. It was not their habit to concede much importance to childhood, and rarely . . . preserved for posterity any of these details of infant life." Desmond, *Newborn Medicine and Society,* xxvii.

Renaissance. Many paintings produced in this era, beginning in the fourteenth century and continuing through the sixteenth century, presented mother and child as noble and spiritual beings worthy of adoration and engendered great public compassion.

Nonetheless, though the relationship of mother and child was revered in the abstract, a very different attitude emerged when it came to specific cases. Thus, from Hellenistic antiquity through the Enlightenment of the seventeenth and eighteenth centuries, huge numbers of parents were known to abandon their children or cause their deaths intentionally. Driven by matters that ranged from illegitimacy and congenital deformity to poverty and war, infants and children were disposed of by parents of every social class. Some infants would be found and fostered out, or sold or given to others; many were left to die.

The practice gave rise to the establishment of foundling homes for unwanted children as early as the thirteenth century, when church-sponsored shelters for children began to flourish throughout Europe. By the eighteenth century, nearly every large European city had a church-sponsored foundling home. With so many children abandoned by desperate parents, admission rates to these homes were staggering.
The Moscow foundling home, established in 1764 by Catherine the Great, accepted up to fourteen thousand abandoned infants per year, many of whom were newly born. In what would become one of the largest hospitals in Paris, the Hospital Des Enfants Trouves, established in the late seventeenth century by Vincent de Paul and the Ladies of Charity, the annual number of admissions in 1772 rose to more than seven thousand infants. By the late 1800s, Italy alone supported well over a thousand foundling homes.[5]

Many of these homes were equipped with a unique architectural feature built into an outer wall and known as a *tour* or *route,* where a baby could be deposited. Designed to ensure infant safety and parental anonymity, the *tour* consisted of a rotating cylindrical box, nearly two feet in diameter, on a turntable. This concave vessel, containing a cradle, faced outside the facility. After placing a baby inside the vessel, the

---

5. Fuchs, *Foundlings and Child Welfare in Nineteenth-Century France,* 10.

donator would ring a bell, alerting the nuns and caretakers within to a new admission. Baby drop-offs were often made in the dead of night by a parent who then swiftly departed.

Many of these foundling homes were converted monasteries; inside, they were often cold, dirty, and damp. Though the homes were established with good intentions, most newborns consigned to them soon died from neglect, malnutrition, or disease. The facilities, aside from religious support, had little to offer. Feeding the newborn was always a challenge, as wet nurses who could supply human milk were often in short supply. Attempts at artificial feeding using "pap boats" proved harmful, only adding to the exorbitant death rate.[6] The children inside the homes were highly vulnerable and susceptible to infectious disease, which spread quickly from one child to the next. Suffering from at the time nontreatable diseases, among them measles, small pox, scarlet fever, cholera, and pertussis (whooping cough), most children succumbed quickly.

The infant mortality rate during this time is illustrated with the following statistics:[7,8]

- Of the recorded 42,674 children admitted to the Moscow foundling home during 1764–98, 37,174, or 87%, died during their stay.

- Of 31,951 children admitted to the Paris foundling home during 1771–77, 25,476, or 80%, died within a year.

- At the Dublin Foundling Asylum, from 1775 to 1796, only 45 children survived out of 10,272—a whopping 99.6 percent mortality rate.

These astronomical infant death rates engendered little surprise or even interest among those who witnessed the horror within the

---

6. *Pap* is a Scandinavian term used for the sound made when a baby opens his mouth for nourishment. A pap boat was a tiny container, resembling a cream pitcher, designed to feed the baby by tipping the feeding, typically a mixture of bread, flour, and water into the mouth. Often contaminated and difficult to clean, the pap boat feeder led to the death of one third of all artificially fed infants.

7. Ransel, *Mothers of Misery*, 48.

8. Garrison, *History of Medicine*, 402.

foundling homes. Some viewed the deaths as acts of natural selection, whereas others perceived them as God's will. These fatalistic views were supported by the reality that there was no existing way to stem the death toll.

Beginning Efforts to Save the Lives of Babies and Children

As society and medicine slowly but steadily evolved, they brought men and women who believed that infants could no longer be ignored.[9] In 1719, during a time properly called the Enlightenment, or the Age of Reason, modern child care would find its rough but essential beginning thanks to an English gentleman named Thomas Coram.

Born in 1668 to a seafaring family, Coram had spent about forty years at sea, much of that time as captain of a merchant vessel.[10] By nature a generous and selfless man, Coram would reportedly seize on opportunities to benefit the public good. Through hard work and dedication, he prospered, eventually retiring with enough wealth to support his modest needs. He finally settled in the port city of Rotherhithe, just southeast of London. As his avocations required, Coram would arrive into London early in the day and return home late at night; in these commutes, he routinely encountered deserted, helpless infants and children who had been callously abandoned. These sightings stirred and enraged him, and as his biographer John Brownlow would note, "He immediately set about inquiring into the probable causes for so outrageous a departure from humanity and affection."[11]

Coram labored for many years, eventually engaging a roster of London notables to sign petitions that led to a royal charter that, in 1739, established the Hospital for the Maintenance and Education of Exposed and Deserted Children, which came to be known as the London Foundling Hospital.[12]

---

9. Rendle-Short and Rendle-Short, *Father of Childcare,* 12.
10. Ibid.
11. Secretary of the hospital Brownlow, *History and Design of the Foundling Hospital,* 63.
12. Ibid., 113–14.

Because the home also served as a symbol of compassion and humanity, it opened to huge public fanfare and received substantial funding from the public. Yet, despite the caring methods employed inside the hospital, its death rates were similar to the rates of other foundling homes of the time. Many infants deposited at the gate did not live long enough to be carried into the wards. Of the 14,934 received, only 4,400 survived and were subsequently adopted.[13]

Brownlow describes the exorbitant death rate:

> It has been truly said that the frail tenure by which an infant holds its life, will not allow of a remitted attention even for a few hours: who therefore, will be surprised, after hearing under what circumstances most of these poor children were left at the hospital gate, that instead of being a protection to the living, the institution became, as it were, a charnel house [burying place] for the dead![14]

Appalled by the staggering infant mortality rate, the board of governors wrote to the Royal College of Physicians requesting help. Responding to the plea was a thirty-seven-year-old physician named William Cadogan (1711–97), who produced a forty-three-page pamphlet titled *An Essay upon Nursing and the Management of Children.*[15]

Advocating simplistic ideas, Cadogan's writings, based in part on his own experience as a father, would usher in a more reasoned approach to child care and new principles of newborn–child management. Written in easy-to-understand language accessible to the lay reader, Cadogan's slim essay would displace centuries of mistaken but socially entrenched infant and child care techniques. Cadogan's little book would also rebuke the widespread use of emetics, purges, and bleeding, all of which were utilized as frontline therapeutic treatments by eighteenth-century

---

13. Ibid., 15–16.
14. Ibid., 15.
15. Rendle-Short and Rendle-Short, *Father of Childcare,* 14–15.

children's physicians. Cadogan would bring to light a much more practical and rational approach to child care, in a period when "mouse dung
dissolved in milk" was an approved treatment for infant constipation.[16]

Among his other rebukes was a caution against the swaddling of
infants into tight bundles, which often included the use of bands to
tie their hands and feet. Advocating the free use of arms and legs to
avoid the risk of deformities, he also dismissed the common notion that
changing babies when needed would "rob them of nourishing juices."
Promoting sound hygienic practices, he advocated the use of clean,
loose-fitting clothing and bedding changed daily. He discredited the
universally held, age-old technique of purging the bowels of meconium
following the infant's delivery. Meconium, the thick, tarry substance
that makes up a baby's first stool, was then thought to cause "fits" if not
evacuated immediately. Honey and butter, syrup of roses, almond oil,
sugared wine, and chicory with rhubarb were among the mendicants
forced down a baby's throat to facilitate the first bowel passage. Cadogan
instead correctly recommended relying on the purgative properties of
the mother's first milk.

He encouraged mothers to breast-feed four times a day for the first
year and to introduce solid foods to the newborn after three months.
He was the first to question the widespread belief that dentition, the
act of teething, was a dangerous condition and the cause of cough, fever, diarrhea, and convulsions, among other ills. He spoke against the
accepted notions that fresh air and cold were injurious to the infant and
instead advised parents to play with their children in the fresh, outdoor
air. With these proposals, Cadogan initiated a fundamentally new way
of caring for the child, changes considered revolutionary at the time.
Because today his principles are part of child-rearing common sense, it
seems inconceivable that they were not always practiced.

Cadogan's focus was the practical management of newborns, and
his advice would offer the first of many major reforms in child care. He
would do more than any other doctor to promote sane and sensible
methods in the rearing of children. His commonsense remedies paved

16. Ibid., 39.

the way to a new understanding of caring for children, and his influence was immense. Printed copies of *An Essay upon Nursing and the Management of Children* would be updated through ten editions and translated into several languages. Widely dispersed among parents and guardians, the essay would become the cornerstone of modern infant and pediatric care literature. Cadogan is now considered the "Father of Child Care."

The Fusion of Artists and Child Care in Europe

Thomas Coram introduced another development in the eighteenth century: to involve London's emerging artistic community in the task of bettering conditions in the foundling home he established. The artists were appalled by the dire conditions in these homes and the way they caused children to suffer and die. The result was that musicians and artists took part, for the first time, in fund-raising activities for these institutions. Among them were William Hogarth, a pioneer in Western sequential art, who, having been touched deeply by the plight of unwanted children, donated some of his most important works to be auctioned to benefit them.

The composer George Frederic Handel performed annual concerts on behalf of the London Foundling Hospital. Several pieces of vocal and instrumental music he composed and performed would, through ticket sales, benefit the hospital foundation. His musical efforts to support the hospital would also lead him to compose the ballad "Blessed Are They That Considereth the Poor and Needy," which came to be known as "The Foundling Hospital Anthem."

Handel's greatest and ongoing contribution involves his most venerated work, *Messiah,* which is full of sacred subject matter and fantastic choral arrangements, designed and drawn from liturgical scripture. Upon his death in 1759, he bequeathed the score, and his organ, to the foundling hospital. The London Foundling Hospital, known today as the Thomas Coram Foundation for Children, continues to use Handel's *Messiah* as its fund-raising centerpiece.[17]

---

17. Brownlow, *History and Design of the Foundling Hospital,* 75.

4

Coming of Age: The Preterm Baby

And can it be that in a world so full and busy,
The loss of one weak creature makes a void in
Any heart, so wide and deep that nothing but the
width and depth of vast eternity can fill it up!
—Charles Dickens, *Dombey and Son*

The London Foundling Hospital was among the European foundling homes to serve as a forerunner to our modern children's hospitals. But the first hospital in the Western world dedicated to the care of sick children, the Hospital Des Enfants Malades (Hospital for Sick Children), was established in Paris in 1802.[18]

At that time, Paris was already distinguishing itself as the epicenter of medical progress, due in part to a neonatal infirmary called the Infirmerie de la Creche, located inside the Paris Foundling Hospice. There the focus was on the care and support of the individual baby and on sick children younger than fifteen years old.

As the nineteenth century progressed, further developments in

---

18. Cone, "L'Hospital Des Enfants-Malades," 670.

child care by the French medical culture would culminate into its most groundbreaking achievement: the first systematic efforts to save the preterm baby. Notably, the evolution of its focus on the well-being of the child would find its impetus not as much in the power of compassion as in a need to expand military might. And so here we confront a supreme paradox: the art of healing can be advanced by the tragedy of wartime casualties.

So it was in France, following the nation's defeat by German-supported forces in the Franco-Prussian War (1870–71); the high casualty rate combined with widespread famine to take a terrible toll on the French population. In addition to France having one of the highest infant mortality rates in Europe (223 deaths out of 1,000 births), a further concern among French leaders was the decline in the birthrate, which was then the lowest in Europe.[19] Germany's birthrate was twice that of France, and French leaders viewed that discrepancy as a military disadvantage because it would lead to diminished French troop levels. In 1891, Jules Simon, a popular French statesman, would proclaim, "France loses a battalion [of soldiers] per year because it lets the infants of the poor die. . . . We let 180,000 infants perish each year. Does France have 180,000 too many that we can allow such assassinations?"[20] Furthermore, national census rates would reveal that deaths in France exceeded births. Driven by the fear of depopulation, French leaders instituted a Commission on Depopulation tasked with finding ways to decrease the infant mortality rate.[21]

Through the influence of the newly established commission, two humane and patriotic obstetricians emerged who would soon change the future of premature infant care: Etienne Stephane Tarnier (1828–97) and Pierre Budin (1846–1907).

Tarnier, educated at the Lycee of Digon, began his internship at the

19. Farr, "Mortality of Children in the Principal States of Europe."

20. Fuchs, *Poor and Pregnant in Paris,* 60; Jules Simon, "De l'initiative privee et de l'etat, en matiere de reformes sociales," in *Conference faite au Grand-Theatre de Bordeaux, November 7, 1891* (Bordeaux, 1892), 19–20.

21. Bolt, *Mortalities of Infancy;* Cone, *History of the Care and Feeding of the Premature Infant,* 15.

Maternite de Paris, a former monastery converted into a women's hospital, which was among the largest maternity hospitals in Europe. Tarnier would rise to become the Maternite's surgeon-in-chief of obstetrics. The industrious physician would revolutionize obstetric aseptic techniques, resulting in the saving of countless mothers from the agony of death by puerperal infections. Historically acknowledged as the "Father of Modern Obstetric Aseptic Technique," his interest thereafter would turn to saving the lives of feeble infants.

On what began as a visit to the Paris Zoo in the summer of 1878, he encountered a poultry incubator exhibition. Inspired by the closed, heated environment containing newly hatched chicks, he contracted with a local instrument maker to construct a similar apparatus for preterm babies.[22] The result was a preterm baby–warming device, or incubator, termed a *couveuse,* or "brooding hen." Commonly viewed as an "external womb," the incubator was designed to mimic the intrauterine environment by maintaining a constant warm and humidified environment, protecting the premature infant against the hazards of the outside environment.

With the use of Tarnier's new incubator, premature infant survival rates inside the Maternite would see a dramatic increase. Not one to rest on his laurels, Tarnier, noting that the more feeble infants were unable to spontaneously take breast milk, would find a solution to feeding smaller and less developed infants. His remedy would come in 1884 in the form of a small, flexible rubber feeding tube to instill milk directly into the infant's stomach, a technique called gavage feeding. Taking its name from the French *gaver,* meaning "to stuff," the new feeding technique would soon become a popular option for the "poor feeder" baby, setting a new medical standard.

During these years, in response to nationalistic fears of depopulation,

---

22. In late-nineteenth-century France, prematurity, or *les prematures,* was sometimes diagnosed not by gestational age but by weight not exceeding twenty-three hundred grams (five pounds). Clarified by the World Health Organization in 1974, *prematurity* is now defined by member nations as less than thirty-seven completed weeks' or 259 days' gestation.

the Paris municipal council would approve funding for the construction of the Pavilion des debiles (pavilion of weaklings) in 1893. Built within the Maternite as a separate structure, the pavilion would be among the most technically advanced special care nurseries of its day. Under the guidance of Professor Tarnier's protégé and eventual successor, Pierre Budin, the pavilion was designed to emphasize the importance of temperature control, feeding, and precautions against infectious disease. The new pavilion would accommodate at least fourteen incubators and contain an independent (steam) heating system, an autoclave for sterilization, and living quarters for its own specially trained staff, including wet nurses.[23] A forerunner to our modern-day neonatal intensive care unit, the Pavilion des debiles would come to symbolize a new phase of infant care.

Having successfully dealt with the health and welfare of feeble infants, Dr. Budin, dismayed at the astounding number of infants who would fail to thrive following birth owing to improper care at home, would establish the first maternal-infant program. Known as the Consultations de Nourissons, the program consisted of an organization of clinics that supervised and educated mothers in the proper care and feeding of infants following hospital discharge. Budin's concepts of infant care would soon set standards that other physicians would replicate throughout France and Europe and, eventually, the United States.

In the course of time, Tarnier's and Budin's mission to save preterm babies and increase the French population would be fulfilled, though not without a human cost. Many of the preterm infant males saved would grow into young, strong men who then were inducted into European wartime activities. Heroic in birth as in death, many of the former preemies would become some of the 1.5 million lives lost on the battlefields of the First World War.

---

23. Baker, *Machine in the Nursery*, 48.

5

The Sanitarians

After nine months of pregnancy a mother is entitled to have her
baby get safe care. To expose her newborn to infection is criminal.
—Bela Schick (1877–1967), Hungarian-born
American pediatrician

Meanwhile, on the other side of the English Channel, public health
officials in England began a major push for public health reform, focusing on preventable sickness and mortality, especially among the poor,
and resulting in sanitary measures that greatly increased public hygiene.
These European health reforms would eventually take hold in America,
where, in the cities, two of every five infants died before reaching their
first birthday.

Beginning Efforts to Save Babies in America

In the 1850s, the *New York Times* began calling attention to the astounding number of infant deaths in America's growing cities. These
calls went largely unheeded until the middle of an unseasonably hot
New York City summer of 1876, when the health department reported
that at least one hundred babies had died in the city each day during a
one-week time frame. A *New York Times* editorial published on July 19,

1876, stated, "There is no more depressing feature about our American Cities than the annual slaughter of little children."[24]

Like other big cities in the United States, New York City had been confronted with a dramatic and sudden increase in population, which produced tons of trash, raw sewage, and filthy debris. Massive amounts of garbage were simply pushed aside or stored on vacant city lots. Over-crowded tenements teeming with the poor and impoverished offered a life of squalor, with no intact sewage systems or running water. Water was bought in by pail and was often contaminated. The tenement con-ditions were compounded by the poor personal hygiene of its many in-habitants, including mothers. Tenement dwellers belonged to the lowest stratum of the urban social class and placed minimal value on cleanli-ness, regular bathing, or the routine changing of clothes. Compounding matters, many of the babies born in these tenements were delivered by midwives who, naively, paid little or no attention to the transmission of contagion to the baby through unwashed hands.

In this era predating automotive technology, pigs, goats, poultry, and horses ran freely in city streets, leaving huge amounts of uncollected manure. The combination of all of these environmental factors, especially over long, hot, and humid summers, provided a perfect breeding ground for the transmission of organisms, notably cholera. The largest number of infant deaths took place within these contaminated and pestilence-filled inner-city environments, often from infectious disease and diarrhea.

From 1850 to 1880, public health officials, inspired by the ear-lier English sanitary campaign, began cleaning up the city in an effort to reduce the high infant mortality rates. These efforts resulted in the development of municipal sewage systems, cleaner water supplies, and more efficient trash and refuse removal systems. Many cities no lon-ger allowed hogs, goats, and cattle to roam at will. Horse owners were pressured to clean up after their mounts; landlords were coerced into cleaning up their buildings. In turn, the infant mortality rate fell from its 1850s high of two out of every five births to one out of every five births by 1880.

---

24. Meckel, *Save the Babies,* 11; *New York Times,* July 19, 1876, p. 4.

Following the implementation of environmental reform within the urban landscape came a second phase of improved public health, beginning around 1880 and lasting through to the 1920s. Its focus was infant feeding. This was essential because public health officials had determined that many infant deaths were related to gastrointestinal disorders (diarrhea) due to contaminated milk supplies and nutrient-deficient breast milk.

Reformers placed emphasis on the quality of feeding and on cleaning up the milk supply. These attempts would eventually lead to the establishment of medical milk commissions whose goal was to guarantee that a germ-free and healthful supply of raw milk was available to the public. Milk sanitarians further supported the cause of decontaminating the existing milk supply through heating the milk followed by rapid cooling. Known as *pasteurization,* the method eliminated many of the microbes responsible for milk contamination. Among sanitarians, the development of pasteurization gained the most support, eventually resulting in mandatory commercial pasteurization of milk in most major American cities.

During this period, it was discovered that many undernourished mothers feared passing on nutrient-deficient breast milk to their babies and were either unwilling or unable to breast-feed. The combination would lead to the development of artificial feeding formulas. The overall result of efforts to clean up and improve the milk supply would mark a dramatic decline in infant death by diarrheal disease, resulting in the reduction of the infant death rate in America.

By 1915, a newly constructed and highly accurate birth registry revealed an infant mortality rate of one death out of every ten births. The 10 percent drop in the mortality rate was an improvement, but much more needed to be done.

Beginning a third phase in the 1920s, public health workers turned their focus to the health of pregnant women. They implemented programs at the community level to educate, monitor, and care for the expectant mother. These efforts included maternal instruction in personal hygiene and nutrition with an emphasis on the importance of breast-feeding. Health care workers provided support throughout the pregnancy up to the time of birth. These programs gained success, spreading throughout America's urban areas. These newly established programs of the era would eventually serve as the foundation of our current-day prenatal care programs, all of which continue to have a positive impact on American maternal–child health.

It was also in the 1920s that concerted efforts were made to save infants born prematurely by placing them in an incubator. American physicians, inspired by European progress in infant care, traveled to Europe for training. One such doctor was an industrious pediatrician by the name of Dr. Julian Hess. On his return home, he designed an electrically heated water-jacketed incubator bed, which was an American version of the French incubator. This important development would lead Dr. Hess, in 1922, to establish America's first premature incubator ward, which was installed in the Sarah Morris Hospital of the Michael Reese Hospital in Chicago. The pioneer premature station was modeled after the Pavilion des debiles of the Paris Maternite. Dr. Hess, a link to our European medical heritage, would also author the first book to deal specifically with prematurity and infant congenital diseases, titled *Premature and Congenitally Diseased Infants.*

The Beginning of Infant Lung Research

Before the close of the 1920s, the path of our story returns to Europe, where it travels deep into the landscape of Switzerland. It is here we meet a spirited young physician by the name of Kurt Von Neergaard, whose work would intersect public health medicine and scientific lung research of the newborn. Neergaard's now famous research on lung function would mark a historic turning point in respiratory care of the newborn.

Born in Schleswig-Holstein, Germany, Neergaard suffered with poor pulmonary health (reports suggest asthma) as a child; eventually, his mother brought him to the famous health center of Davos, a mountaintop sanatorium high in the Swiss Alps. The fresh air quality of Davos, the highest point in all of Europe, was then considered a valued therapeutic treatment for pulmonary health problems and was often recommended as a destination for lung disease patients.

Neergaard remained in Switzerland, became a citizen, and graduated from the University of Zurich. Although he was a physician, Neergaard did not pursue patient care and instead chose to experiment with lung function. In 1922, he moved to Basel, where he began to study lung elasticity and airway flow resistance in the normal, asthmatic, and emphysemic lung. Of these experiments, those that would influence Neergaard's thinking the most were his studies on lung elasticity. Working with healthy, excised porcine lungs, he concluded that there existed an interfacial tension between the alveolar (singular: alveolus) air and the membrane covering it, and this boundary was largely responsible for the lungs' elastic recoil. He described this wet lining inside the air sacs of the lung, or alveoli, as *surface tension,* a force not unlike the taunt surface of a trampoline, where a downward force is compensated by an upward one. Neergaard clearly realized that surface tension acting on the alveoli gave them the ability to expand and contract. Neergaard would be the first to suggest in scientific literature a connection between surface tension and the elastic properties of the lungs.

Neergaard published his now classic paper in German.[25] Medical discoveries then traveled slowly, and the barrier of a foreign language was difficult to overcome. For these reasons, nearly a quarter century passed before those few in the evolving field of lung studies took note of Neergaard's discovery. Neergaard, though aware of the importance of his findings, made no further inquiries to build on them. Perhaps lacking clear insight into the future or simply losing interest, Neergaard dropped his lung studies and his hypothesis, which time would reveal to be a major discovery. His follow-through could conceivably have saved thousands of infant lives, including that of Patrick Bouvier Kennedy. Nevertheless, Neergaard purportedly changed pursuits and, in the 1930s, a period characterized by catastrophic changes in European

---

25. The title in English is "New Notions on a Fundamental Principle of Respiratory Mechanics: The Retractile Force of the Lung, Dependent on the Surface Tension in the Alveoli."

culture, began to write prolifically on the relationship between medicine and society.

Neergaard's groundbreaking findings were an expansion of earlier research into human lungs by the German worker K. Hochheim. As early as 1903, Hochheim began investigating the causes of airway disease inside the lungs of infants who died shortly after birth. Using newly developed microscopic staining techniques enabling him to see the unique architecture of the alveoli, Hochheim noted the existence of a peculiar appearing, glassy membrane inside the baby lung. He would be the first to correctly describe and name the *hyaline membrane* from the Greek *hyal,* "glass," and the Latin *ine,* "chemical substance." Originally published in German, Hochheim's paper would have the same fate as Neergaard's, its contents going unrecognized for decades.

Notwithstanding, sixty years later, following the death of Patrick Bouvier Kennedy from hyaline membrane disease, the strange term would find its way outside of a small circle of scientists and become a major part of the social lexicon. Claiming thousands of babies per year, HMD would eventually come to be known as respiratory distress syndrome.

6

Naming Respiratory Distress Syndrome

They do certainly give very strange and newfangled names to diseases.
—Plato, *The Republic*

Midway through the American twentieth century, reports claimed that premature birth was the primary cause of infant deaths in the first year. Of those infants, most would die from a lung disease bought on by the lungs' prematurity. The premature lung disease causing the baby's severe shortness of breath was then called by many names.

In the present day, respiratory distress syndrome, or RDS, is the favored name for respiratory distress of the newborn, and for the sake of consistency, I use this term throughout the book. The naming of RDS is a story worth telling and stands as a prime example of how naming a disease can be a long, drawn-out process. Putting a name to a disease is an extremely important undertaking because it is the first major step in gathering resources to fight the malady.

It is worth noting that in Patrick Bouvier Kennedy's time, RDS was more often called hyaline membrane disease, or HMD. As noted earlier, the hyaline membrane is the glassy chemical substance seen inside the alveolar capillary membrane through the microscopic lens of the pathologist doing a postmortem examination, or autopsy, of the infant lung. And so the term hyaline membrane disease describes the *scientific makeup* of the malady.

Conversely, RDS takes its name from the Latin *respiratio,* "breathing," *distringere,* "distress by physical suffering," and *syndrome,* from the Greek roots, *syn* and *drom,* indicating "symptoms linked to a disease." Taken together, the name "respiratory distress syndrome" beautifully describes the stricken babies' most outstanding clinical feature, which is difficulty in breathing.

During the first half of the twentieth century, very few doctors understood the mechanism of RDS, and fewer yet could explain the disease. For this reason, among others, by the early 1950s, no fewer than nine terms were invented to help diagnose and explain the puzzling lung syndrome now called RDS:[26]

1. myelin formation in the lungs

2. congenital aspiration pneumonia

3. asphyxial membrane

4. desquamative anaerosis

5. congenital alveolar dysplasia

6. vernix membrane

7. hyaline membrane

8. hyaline-like membrane

9. hyaline atelectasis

Given the large number of names, diagnosticians continued to grope for a more suitable term. By the mid-1950s, three more names had been added to the growing list of terms: idiopathic respiratory distress syndrome of the newborn, pulmonary syndrome of the newborn, and, finally, respiratory distress syndrome.

Because there was no universal agreement about what to name the

---

26. Tran and Anderson, "Hyaline-Like Membranes Associated with Disease of the Newborn Lungs."

disease, a conference was held in 1959, in Montreal, to formally name it.[27] In attendance were thirty prominent pediatricians and pathologists. Among those participating were several profiled in this book: James Drorbaugh, Clement Smith, Mary Ellen Avery, Virginia Apgar, and Peter Grunewald. After a heated discussion, a vote was taken. The result, which served only to frustrate its organizers, was as follows: fifteen voted to name it "idiopathic respiratory distress syndrome of the newborn," four voted to call it "pulmonary syndrome of the newborn," and coming in third were three votes for "hyaline membrane disease"! The remainder did not vote at all, presumably confused as to what to name the disease.

Knowledge of the infant lung disease slowly advanced, and by the early 1960s, many names were displaced in favor of only two: hyaline membrane disease and respiratory distress syndrome.

In the late 1980s, when I began practicing in the NICU, one would occasionally encounter older NICU staff who spoke of or wrote HMD instead of RDS. Nowadays, it's rare to hear the term HMD or to see it written on a patient chart.

I recently conducted an informal survey inside the NICU where I practice. Targeting a younger group of nurses and respiratory care practitioners whose educational backgrounds encompassed extensive education in RDS, I discovered, surprisingly, that many had never even heard of HMD.

America's Hard Years

The American Academy of Pediatrics (AAP) was founded in 1930, during the Great Depression. Three years later came the establishment of the pediatric specialty certification by the AAP. This was the beginning of pediatrics as its own scholarly discipline, allowing medical doctors to emerge from training as board-certified pediatricians. The 1930s also saw a decline in newborn infections and diarrhea, all thanks to cleaner environments, better personal hygiene, and the widespread use of breast milk. Notwithstanding, it was during this decade that newborn deaths by prematurity began to exceed those caused by infection.

27. Rudolph and Smith, "Idiopathic Respiratory Distress of the Newborn."

Highlighting the seriousness of the matter, the AAP passed a resolution in 1935 defining the premature infant as one who weighs twenty-five hundred grams—five and half pounds—or less, regardless of gestational age. Classifying and naming a specific type of baby needing special attention was a monumental step toward organizing social and scientific forces in support of the premature infant.

The Dionne Quintuplets

The event that familiarized mainstream society with the preterm infant began in the wee hours of May 28, 1934, in a small, remote cabin on the outskirts of the Canadian village of Corbeil, Ontario. It was then and there that five premature baby girls became the first successful quintuplet delivery in recorded medical history. They would be known as the Dionne Quintuplets.

The astonishing delivery began shortly before Dr. Allan Defoe, a local obstetrician, entered the Dionnes' small, four-room farmhouse. Contacted earlier to attend what reportedly would be a twin birth, by the time he'd arrived, two babies had already been born, and the other three appeared within half an hour. Dr. Dafoe estimated the total weight of all five as not being more than the weight of a single large, born-at-term baby. He was also aware that no quintuplets were ever known to have survived. Initially, the babies were moistened with olive oil and crammed into a butcher's basket, which was set on two chairs directly in front of an open oven. Every two hours, warm water was dropped into their mouths using a medicine dropper. For the first days, they were fed with thirty to sixty drops of a mixture of cow's milk and corn syrup.[28]

To everyone's surprise, the babies not only survived but were active and showed few signs of distress. Once news of the births was published in the local paper, word spread quickly throughout Canada and the United States. Soon nurses volunteered to help care for the infants. Desperately needed incubators were donated and flown in from Chicago. Responding to the extra need for mother's milk, nursing mothers within easy traveling distance volunteered to wet nurse. Anticipating the

---

28. Berton, *Dionne Years,* 38.

heat of the upcoming summer, refrigerators were supplied to keep the milk cold. Clothing, linen, and blankets arrived, shipped from distant cities by kindly strangers. Specialist volunteers from around the United States and Canada offered assistance to Dr. Defoe, free of charge. In the small Dionne home, where five siblings and two parents were already living, space became cramped. It soon became evident that, for the babies to survive, they would need the support and care that only a modern hospital could provide. But there was no nearby hospital and the quintuplets were too fragile to be moved. The Canadian Red Cross stepped in and built a large nursery, called the Dafoe Hospital, for the Dionne Quintuplets. Built directly across the road from the original Dionne homestead, the hospital would include nine permanent staff, including three policemen, to accommodate the needs of and protect these five special babies.

During the dark period of the Great Depression, the quintuplets became a phenomenon, perhaps a light to a society in need of hope. *Time* magazine would call them the "greatest news-picture story" ever told.[29] Hundreds of thousands of visitors, drawn from all parts of the world, came to get a glimpse of them. Corbeil soon became a tourist destination and took on the atmosphere of a county fair. When the infants were a few months old, during the summer season, visitors exceeded an estimated seven thousand daily. Hundreds of parked cars filled the area around the Dionne hospital. Every available source for overnight accommodations was exhausted, and spare rooms within fifty miles were taken up. Many visitors had to be turned away.

In their first few days of life, the babies had been weighed using a potato scale. All five weighed a total of just thirteen pounds five ounces. On June 4, roughly five weeks after they were born, their weights ranged from two pounds six ounces to eleven pounds ten ounces. Yet, by the time the Dionne sisters reached five years of age, the weight and size of each was equal to that of an average five-year-old.[30]

The Dionne Quintuplets legitimized medical attempts to save

---

29. Ibid., 16.
30. Thornton, *Country Doctor,* 95.

premature infants and gave hope to many that babies born extremely premature and with abnormally low birth weights can survive.

Incubator-Baby Sideshows

In the midst of the sensational Dionne Quintuplet births, the Chicago World's Fair of 1933–34 was in full swing. Titled "Chicago's Century of Progress Exposition," the theme of the fair was technological innovation with the motto "Science Finds, Industry Applies, Man Conforms." Inside the international symposium, a visitor would encounter one of the strangest events in the history of newborn care: the Incubator-Baby Sideshows. Among the other sideshow attractions, which ostensibly included a bearded lady, a fat man, a skinny man, and Siamese twins, were a number of standing incubators containing live preterm babies.

The person responsible for the Incubator-Baby Sideshows was the creative and resourceful Dr. Martin Couney (1870–1950), a specialist in the care of premature infants and famously known as the "incubator doctor." Born in France, Couney studied under the tutelage of Pierre Budin at the Maternite. Years earlier, while in Europe, Couney had displayed incubators and infants at the request of Dr. Budin, who asked him to present the newly modified Tarnier incubator at the 1896 World Exposition in Berlin. Budin's intent was to promote the new incubator technology, though Couney decided that live preterm babies would add extra sizzle to the exhibit. The exhibit, the first of its kind, was called "Kinderbrutanstalt," or "Child Hatchery," and became wildly successful among fairgoers.

In the hope of duplicating his success in America, in 1898, Couney left Europe for the World's Fair in Omaha, Nebraska. Dubbed the Omaha Trans-Mississippi Exposition, the goal of the fair was to showcase turn-of-the-century developments of the entire West. There Couney would set up his first incubator display on American soil. Among his objectives were to showcase the newest incubator technology utilizing the appeal of live preterm infants and, in the process, educate the public about the plight of the preterm baby.

Oddly enough, Couney had a connection to the Dionne

Quintuplets, who were born while he was exhibiting his incubator show at the Chicago World's Fair in May 1934. Looking to capitalize on the Dionnes' story, Randolph Hearst, the newspaper baron, offered to send Couney from the Chicago fair to Corbeil accompanied by a reporter and photographer. Despite Mr. Hearst's offer of a generous fee, Couney declined, saying his responsibility was to the thirty babies under his care at the Chicago fair. Couney also mentioned to Hearst his concern that there would be no natural gas to heat his incubators in rural Canada. Couney would later confide to a colleague that he did not believe the quints would survive, putting him in fear of a highly publicized failure.[31]

Before Couney departed Chicago for the East Coast, he donated the sideshow incubators to Julian Hess at the Sarah Morris Hospital of the Michael Reese Hospital. He also donated to the city of Chicago the ambulance used to transport his incubator babies from the hospital to the fairgrounds. Containing a modified Hess incubator in the rear, the ambulance would become the very first premature infant transport vehicle in the United States.

The incubator shows continued while public and medical enthusiasm came and went, and by the end of the 1940s, the exhibitions fizzled out. It remains uncertain if Couney was more of a circus entertainer or a fundamental link between French and American neonatal medicine. What is certain is that the incubator sideshows are one of the more controversial and bizarre chapters in the history of newborn care.

The 1940s

In the 1940s, the infant death rate in the United States remained abysmally high, claiming approximately forty-seven babies out of every one thousand born alive. The decade would see many steps taken to further the care of the newborn, though few would exceed the value of the first American textbook on neonatology, authored by Dr. Clement Smith of the Harvard Medical School and titled *Physiology of the Newborn Infant*.

This comprehensive treatise was the first to describe the embryology, physiology, and cardiopulmonary systems of the newborn. Its

---

31. Silverman, "Incubator-Baby Side Shows."

publication in 1946 allowed specialized knowledge to become available to a widespread clinical audience, while raising standards of newborn care. Dr. Smith would later become director of the Neonatal Research Lab at the Boston Lying-in Hospital, where, in 1963, his team would play a significant role in the care of Patrick Bouvier Kennedy.[32] Today, Dr. Smith is regarded as a pioneering force in neonatology.

Meanwhile, newborn lung research continued at an agonizingly slow pace. In the early 1940s, Peter Grunewald, an anatomist and embryologist trained in Vienna, arrived in the United States, where he soon found employment as a pediatric and developmental pathologist in the Department of Pathology at New York's Kings County Hospital. He studied the alveoli, the microscopic air sacs inside the lungs, of autopsied infants who had succumbed to lung disease. In 1947, unaware of Neergaard's earlier work, he duplicated the methods of the Swiss pioneer and concluded that "surface tension is a major factor in the resistance of the lung of the newborn to aeration."[33] Grunewald further suggested that atelectasis, or collapse of the alveoli in newborns, might be avoided if a surface active agent were added to the air or oxygen the infant inhaled.[34]

The close of the 1940s would bring about many new beginnings in newborn care. Among them were the first clinical use of penicillin, advances in the treatment of hemolytic disease, and intravenous infusion of electrolyte therapy and fluids. Also during the decade, cardiac catheterization for the diagnosis of congenital heart disease would lead to the first surgical interventions and successes in infant cardiac care.

The 1940s would also see more extensive treatment of the preterm baby and the indiscriminate and highly regrettable use of 100 percent oxygen. Utilized as a frontline treatment strategy for the preterm baby in respiratory distress, oxygen therapy would result in the blinding of thousands of premature babies.[35] National statistical databases in the

---

32. Dr. Smith was vacationing in Europe when Patrick Kennedy was admitted to Boston Children's Hospital. Will Cochran, personal interview with the author.

33. Comroe, *Retro Spectro Scope,* 150.

34. Ibid.

35. Stevie Wonder, the American singer and songwriter, born premature, was among those blinded by exposure to an oxygen-enriched environment.

1940s would also confirm prematurity as the leading cause of infant death. Records show that one-half of the babies born premature died within the first twenty-four hours, a statistic correlating with death by RDS.

The early 1950s would see many new developments in newborn care. Leading the way was Dr. Virginia Apgar, an anesthesiologist who, in 1951, developed a newborn scoring system to be applied within the first five to ten minutes of a baby's life. The newly configured Apgar score would encourage delivery room personnel to focus attention on the baby in the first minutes of life. Based on a simple five-point grading system, the score encompassed the activity of heart rate, respiratory effort, reflexes, muscle tone, and skin color, allowing delivery room personnel to instantly recognize when immediate help was needed.

Other major strides in newborn premature care were engineering improvements of the newborn incubator to meet physician requests for adjustable oxygen concentrations and improved visibility in the incubator. A new glass enclosure allowed direct observation of breathing patterns of the unwrapped baby while reducing the newborns exposure to the often-cool temperature outside the incubator.

In the meantime, the study of hyaline membranes, and their association to newborn lung disease, slowly gained momentum. In 1953, doctors studying RDS would begin to correlate its progression with chest X-rays. Babies at risk for developing RDS would be divided into three groups: premature infants, infants delivered by cesarean section, and infants born of diabetic mothers. Though the mysterious disease targeted these groups, it was not understood what caused hyaline membranes to form in the lungs, preventing oxygen from entering the bloodstream. Scientists exploring other causes suggested that the membranes were created by hormonal imbalances stemming from the mother, by the inhalation of amniotic fluid into the lungs, or by ingestion of blood into the lungs associated with C-section.

In the 1950s, there would also be various attempts to treat RDS, and one contraption designed to do just that was called the Bloxam air lock.[36] This complex mechanical device consisted of a closed chamber into which the baby was placed. Designed to mimic in utero contractions, the machine soon fell out of favor. The air lock would be followed by a series of ill-fated attempts to treat RDS, though few would exceed the popularity and longevity of the mist nebulizer. Developed to relieve RDS, water-based mist treatments were infused into the isolette, producing a fog so thick that, according to witnesses, "you couldn't even see the baby," and the "nurses had to place their stethoscope inside on the infant's chest to make sure he was still alive."[37]

In 1953, a new drug called Alevaire would emerge that would be touted as a cure for RDS. The detergent-based drug would be added to a base water solution for misting into the isolette. Following controlled trials in 1955, the medication proved ineffective.[38] Another attempt to treat RDS in the mid-1950s was by a procedure called *sternal traction,* which is accomplished by suturing a line into the top of the baby's chest wall and attaching it to a rigid overhead structure. Sternal traction was utilized on RDS babies whose every inhaled breath was so deep the chest appeared to meet the spine. The traction procedure was thought to stabilize the babies' chest wall. The then popular technique, though well intentioned, would, fortunately, soon fall out of favor.

Surfactant Research

During the 1950s, a small group of lung researchers were adding to a better understanding of scientific investigations that later would help explain the pathophysiology of Patrick Kennedy's death. Once again, we encounter Dr. Peter Grunewald, teaching lung physiology now at the Johns Hopkins University in Baltimore. Dr. Grunewald was recognized as one of a handful of researchers in the world who could knowledgeably discuss HMD, and it was at Hopkins that he would influence a young, aspiring medical student by the name of Mary Ellen Avery. Soon

---

36. Silverman, *Retrolental Fibroplasia,* 72.
37. Will Cochran, interview with the author, Lancaster, Massachusetts, November 12, 2012.
38. Silverman, *Retrolental Fibroplasia,* 73.

to be a major figure in HMD research, Avery's story is worth reviewing.

As a young physician, Avery, like her predecessor Neergaard, would be diagnosed with a pulmonary ailment. A few months after receiving her MD from Johns Hopkins in 1952, she was diagnosed with tuberculosis during a routine physical exam. Although asymptomatic, she was prescribed streptomycin and directed to the Trudeau Sanatorium in upstate New York for a year of bed rest. Following only a few days there, her mind raced contemplating the efficacy of the established tuberculosis treatment. How would bed rest help the lungs, she wondered, and what about the drug she was taking? She soon checked out of the facility and continued her convalescence at her parents' home in Moorestown, New Jersey. During this time, realizing she hadn't a clue as to how the established tuberculosis treatment worked, she began corresponding with a friend at Hopkins, Richard Riley, a pulmonary expert and teacher. Following her enquiries to Riley for help in understanding bed rest and the resting lung, she was struck by the near-absolute lack of information on the subject. Intrigued by the scarcity of information regarding pulmonary mechanics in addition to her own lung ailment, she was led to become a pediatrician specializing in lung disease. In 1954, fully recuperated she returned to John Hopkins Hospital, where under the tutelage of the pathologist Peter Gruenwald, would be deeply influenced by his teachings on lung mechanics.

At about this time in the 1950s, also known as the post–World War II era, small notice was given to military research laboratories established in Great Britain, Canada, and the United States. In yet another example of how scientists would coax unintended medicinal–humanistic value from warfare research, researchers began to study the effects of poisonous inhaled gases used in wartime activities. The military would use these findings with the goal of preventing, diagnosing, and treating those victimized by wartime gases. The studies would begin a small revolution in respiratory physiology.

For example, at the Chemical Defense Experimental Laboratory in Porton Down, England, Richard Pattle, a laboratory employee, researched the effect of war gases, notably phosgene, on the lining of the lungs. Pattle, educated as a physicist, noted the remarkable ability of the lung to withstand warfare gas agents, suggesting the alveoli must be covered with a lining allowing for a low surface tension. He further observed that a thin film within the alveoli, responsible for shielding the lung against damage, was produced within the lung itself. His conclusion was that the absence of a thin, liquid film covering the lung's air sacs might play a part in alveolar collapse, suggesting in turn that its deficiency might be the cause of the hyaline membrane inside the infant lung.

Meanwhile, across the Atlantic, deep into the reaches of Canada, with work supported by the Canadian Chemical Warfare Laboratories, Charles Macklin discovered remarkable characteristics of the surface lining of the lungs and would become the first to propose the existence of lung surfactant.

Simultaneously, our scene shifts southward to the Army Chemical Corps Medical Research Laboratories in Edgewood, Maryland, where we meet a newly minted MD by the name of Dr. John Clements. Employed by the army as a researcher, Clements arrived at Edgewood in 1950.

Clements's initial assignments in Edgewood were twofold. One was to study how nerve gas would damage the lungs; the other was to help supervise military contracts to universities, among them one given to the Harvard School of Public Health. In the course of his work traveling to Harvard, Clements would meet Jeremiah Mead, then head of the Department of Physiology at the Harvard School of Public Health, and Edward Radford, also in Mead's laboratory. The small group of lung investigators in the Harvard lab were then known as the most knowledgeable lung investigators in the United States. His personal acquaintance and discussions with these veteran lung pros inspired Clements to involve himself in lung research.

Meanwhile, Edward Radford, at the Harvard School of Public Health, was acquainted with Neergaard's work and, having calculated the surface area of the lungs' alveoli, had to assume that a surface tension existed, as Neergaard had posited nearly a quarter century earlier.

Radford concluded that the surface tension was large and the alveolar surface area small, which, if true, would mean the alveoli are coated with a film (surfactant) to keep the air sacs from collapsing.

Then, in 1955, two important things happened. First, an anesthesiologist by the name of Elwyn Brown was assigned to Clements's lab.[39] The other matter of consequence was an article by Richard Pattle that appeared in the journal *Nature* on the subject of the alveoli.[40] In his landmark paper, Pattle proposed that the alveoli owed their (soap-bubble-like) stability not to body fluid outside the lung but to a substance produced by the lung itself. Prattle's article shed new light on Radford's experiment, which suggested the existence of a film that kept the alveoli from collapsing. Pattle's article and Radford's experiment began discourse between Clements and Brown on the matter. Brown, who had been trained in chemical engineering and physical chemistry, would devise new and improved experimental methods duplicating Radford's experiments. The successful outcome of Brown's experiments would also lead him to conclude that surface tension in the alveoli suggested the presence of a film that worked to keep the alveoli open. Brown and Clements would collaborate for two more years, further refining proof of a liquid film that kept the alveoli open and prevented them from collapsing.

Ultimately, Clements would determine that the very thin, foamy film coating the lung sacs does play a primary role in keeping the lungs' alveoli open. The finding would also lead Clements to put a name to the film coating the alveoli, coining the term *pulmonary surfactant,* from "surface active agent."

In 1957, in a paper titled "Surface Tension of Lung Extracts," Clements would publish his important findings on surface tension, though the paper would stimulate little interest outside the small group of enthusiasts involved in lung studies.[41]

By the late 1950s, the background research was completed for

---

39. Dr. Brown is also known as a pioneer in formulating modern CPR technique.
40. Pattle, "Properties, Function and Origin of the Alveolar Lining Layer."
41. Clements, "Surface Tension of Lung Extracts."

understanding the lungs' alveolar lining and its role in the deaths of untold numbers of premature infants. What was needed was an imaginative, well-trained, energetic pediatrician able to put all this information together, and that person would be Mary Ellen Avery.

We pick up the thread of Avery's life in 1957, when she was drawn to the Harvard School of Public Health to study respiratory physiology and newborn medicine. Attracted by the reputation of Jeremiah Mead's research in infant pulmonology, she began a fellowship in Mead's laboratory in the Department of Physiology under Dr. James Whittenberger. Working as a pediatrician by day, under the tutelage of Clement Smith, at the Boston Lying-in Hospital (across the street), she watched helplessly as babies died from RDS. In the evening, back across the street in Mead's lab, she reviewed postmortem lung specimans obtained from the Lying-in pathologist of infants who had succumbed to RDS. Mixing bedside observation with medical research, she discovered in the infant lung the absence of foam, a characteristic of surfactant, contributing to the conclusion that the lungs were deficient in surfactant.

At this time, a serendipitous meeting would take place, one that would be responsible for taking hard research out of the lab and into the newborn nursery. James Whittenberger, director of the Meads lab and John Clements's advisor, brought news to Avery of a recent article by Clements proposing a dynamic method of measuring surface tension using a modified laboratory apparatus called a Wilhelmy balance, which was a surface film balance scale. During the 1957 Christmas season, Avery visited Clements's lab, where he demonstrated that the contraption could measure the surface tension of lung extracts. Avery reportedly stated later that "that was her Christmas present from Clements."

Avery returned to Boston, where she and Mead devised their own modified apparatus comparing the lungs of infants who had died both with and without having RDS. Through those observations, they noted that infants who died but did not have RDS had foam, or surfactant, in their lungs, whereas babies who expired because of RDS were foam deficient.

Avery and Mead postulated that a lack of foam, or surfactant, in babies' lungs might be the cause of RDS. The observations and research would lead them to publish a paper in 1959 titled "Surface Properties in Relation to Atelectasis and Hyaline Membrane Disease."[42] This now famous paper would be the first to show that pulmonary surfactant was deficient in the lungs of babies dying from RDS. Clements, echoing Avery, would remark, "That was their [Avery and Mead's] Christmas present to me."[43]

The startling scientific discovery, Nobel Prize–worthy in scope, gained little attention beyond the small group of scientists involved in infant lung studies. Snugly ensconced in the optimism of a postwar culture and cast against the appeal of circuses and spectator sports, society had little reason to glance at something so unappealing as infant lung disease. America, a culture in full stride, with many of its great problems left far behind, would receive a great blow in 1963 with the death of Patrick Bouvier Kennedy.

In the early 1960s, America's dramatically rising population was approaching 200 million and averaging well over ten thousand births *per day*. This staggering birthrate would be accompanied by a corresponding rise in infant mortality, as twenty-six babies died out of every one thousand live births.

The leading cause of these deaths was premature birth accompanied by RDS. Clearly, if this deadly condition could be treated in the preterm infant population, infant mortality rates would decrease dramatically. This was a compelling reason to find a way to treat RDS.

As we have seen, this scientific saga was propelled by a miniscule group of remarkably creative scientists numbering fewer than a dozen. What they shared was a devotion to the study of the infant lung; the common thread of their findings is that they were largely ignored by the many. But then came summer 1963, and the very lung disease they were beginning to understand would be the primary cause of death of a baby born to the president of the United States.

---

42. Avery and Mead, "Surface Properties in Relation to Atelectasis and Hyaline Membrane Disease."
43. Clements, "Lung Surface Tension and Surfactant."

We may now see that the evolution of newborn lung research was very slow and tedious. This would change with Patrick's birth and death, which prompted an abrupt upward shift in newborn research and, in so doing, drew the entire discipline into the modern age.

7

Patrick's Birth

Everyone is a hero at birth, where he undergoes a tremendous
physical and psychological transformation, from the condition
of a little water creature living in a realm of amniotic fluid into
an air breathing mammal which ultimately will be standing.
—Otto Rank, *The Myth of the Birth of the Hero*

In the summer of 1963, Jacqueline Bouvier Kennedy was pregnant for
the fifth time. Beginning in late spring of that year, numerous precau-
tionary measures had been arranged in the event of an obstetric emergency. The baby was due in September, to be delivered at the Walter
Reed Medical Center in Washington, D.C., but because Mrs. Kennedy
was spending much of her last trimester on Cape Cod's Squaw Island,
special accommodations had been installed for her at the hospital of the
nearby Otis Air Force Base.

These quarters were housed in Building 3703, which had previously served as an office for the president when he was vacationing in
Hyannis Port at the Kennedy compound.

Refurbished by air force personnel at a cost of five thousand dollars
(nearly forty thousand in today's dollars), the prefab military structure
was one among a row of structures that housed the nursing staff. Containing eight air-conditioned rooms spread out over some twenty-one

hundred square feet of living space, the extensive remodel of the interior contrasted with the building's drab outer appearance. Designed to transition Mrs. Kennedy into an environment that felt like home, the space was divided into four bedrooms, an ample-sized sitting room, and a nursery. Each of the rooms was painted an off white with green tile, paneled in light plywood with matching brown and white drapes. Topping it off were furnishings purchased from Jordan Marsh, an upscale Boston department store. The president had been unaware of the extent of the remodel until he came upon an article in the *Washington Post* that provided a detailed description of the lodgings, including its hefty cost to taxpayers. Jackie's elaborate birthing suite, mocked by the press, would rapidly escalate into a political liability and embarrassment for the president.

Aside from that unexpectedly thorny matter, preparations had gone smoothly. As early as June, JFK's personal doctor, Dr. Janet Travell, was stationed inside special quarters on the air force base premises. As an added safeguard, Jackie's personal obstetrician, Dr. John Walsh, was ensconced in a house not far from the Kennedy's rented home on Squaw Island.

JFK had always wanted to have many children, and Jackie had tried to comply. Her first pregnancy, in 1955, the year they were married, had resulted in a miscarriage. The following year, at thirty weeks' pregnant, she suffered severe cramps and bleeding and was rushed to a hospital in Newport, Rhode Island. There doctors performed an emergency cesarean section, but the baby, Arabella, was born dead (stillborn). Her third pregnancy, in 1957, resulted in the cesarean birth of a healthy, full-term baby girl, Caroline. Her fourth pregnancy, in 1960, ended with early labor and another C-section to deliver John Jr., born four weeks premature and weighing six pounds three ounces. Though reported to be in satisfactory health, John Jr. had initial breathing difficulties that also required a period of incubation.

Now, as they readied for a third child, it had been decided that, if the baby were a boy, he would be named after JFK's immigrant grandfather, Patrick, while his middle name would be Bouvier, in honor of Jackie's father.

August 7, 1963, was a clear, cool morning on Squaw Island. The house, Jackie's favorite hideout, sat close to the sea and thus still nearer to the first lady's heart. Furnished simply in early American fashion, upholstered and straight-backed chairs surrounded interspersed tables, accompanied by separate bookcases that lent a touch of elegance to its interior. On the yellow-painted walls hung landscape and seascape paintings, many by Jackie's own hand.

Jackie, under strict orders from her obstetrician to take it easy, had limited the day's activities to taking five-year-old Caroline and two-year-old John Jr. to their daily horseback riding lessons in nearby Osterville. The children piled into the backseat of an open convertible driven by Secret Service agent Paul Landis and soon arrived at the stables where their ponies were kept. While they scrambled out of the car, Jackie remained in the front seat suddenly paralyzed by acute pains in her back and stomach. Suspecting that she might once again be going into early labor, she told Agent Landis to gather the children and return home immediately. It was 11:00 A.M. when Ensign George Dalton, stationed inside the mobile trailer in the rear of the Kennedy's rented house that served as headquarters for the Secret Service, received a call from Agent Landis. Dalton immediately summoned Dr. Walsh and then alerted the hospital at Otis Air Force Base that the baby appeared to be arriving ahead of schedule. This well-rehearsed emergency notification set into motion the careful preparations for Jackie's emergency admission to the hospital, the first of which was immediate dispatch of an air force helicopter to bring her to the hospital at Otis.

When Jackie arrived at the Squaw Island house, Dr. Walsh was already there, as were Dr. Travell and Mary Gallagher, Jackie's personal secretary. Jackie exclaimed, "I think I'm going to have the baby!"[44] Dr. Walsh's hasty examination revealed she was right. "Dr. Walsh, you've just got to get me to the hospital on time! I don't want anything to happen to this baby," she said. Dr. Walsh, himself unable to calm down, patted her hand, assuring her, "We'll have you there in plenty of time."[45]

---

44. Gallagher, *My Life with Jacqueline Kennedy*, 286.
45. Ibid., 287.

Caroline and John Jr. were quickly consigned to the care of their vigilant Secret Service agents. Moments later, Dr. Walsh, Jackie, and Mary Gallagher stepped onto the lawn and boarded the air force helicopter that would airlift them to the Otis hospital. It was 11:28 A.M. when the chopper lifted for the twenty-mile flight.

Jacqueline Kennedy was a determinedly private person, a woman who steadfastly kept her innermost thoughts to herself. But no one could doubt where those thoughts had traveled when she turned to her doctor again and pleaded, "This baby mustn't be born dead."[46]

Clearly she was thinking of Arabella, her first-born child, who had lain, these past seven years, in a Newport, Rhode Island, cemetery, beneath a stone marked with a single word: "Daughter."

By the time Jackie's helicopter was aloft, JFK was in the Oval Office, wrapping up after his second appointment of the day: a meeting with Dr. Neftali Ponce-Miranda, the foreign minister of Ecuador, who had left at 11:37 A.M.[47]

Prior to that, the president had attended the conference for the Citizens Committee for a Nuclear Test Ban. It was presided over by the committee's chief, James Wadsworth, former U.S. delegate to the United Nations.

By then, Dr. Travell had hurried to the Secret Service trailer behind the Kennedy house. There, she called Jerry Behn, the agent in charge of the White House, who relayed the news to Evelyn Lincoln, the president's secretary. It was 11:43 when Mrs. Lincoln rushed into the Oval Office to tell the president that Jackie had gone into premature labor.

Within moments, at the president's command, the Secret Service was mapping out the swiftest way to transport him to Otis.

At 11:48 A.M., the helicopter carrying Mrs. Kennedy touched down at Otis Air Force Base, which had been closed to all but authorized personal in anticipation of her arrival. She was placed in a waiting ambulance and rushed to the hospital, where three healthy airmen who

---

46. Ibid., 286.
47. All times are as recorded in the official White House appointment book, http://microsites.jfklibrary.org/presidentsdesk/august 7-9 1963.

shared her blood type (A1 Rh positive) and had been chosen weeks before were standing by to donate blood should a transfusion be required.

At 11:52 A.M., twenty-seven minutes after Dr. Travell's phone call, the president's air force helicopter lifted off the south lawn of the White House for the brief flight to Andrews Air Force Base. He was accompanied by Mrs. Lincoln, two Secret Service agents, his military aide General McHugh, and Pamela Turnure, receptionist and secretary to the president. Also on board was the White House press secretary, Pierre Salinger, who had already issued a press release about the impending birth.

At 12:03 P.M., they landed at Andrews only to discover that one of the president's personal air force jets was en route to Moscow, carrying a group of nuclear test ban negotiators, while the other was temporarily out of commission. A third presidential jet, duly equipped with the complex communications setup that accompanies the chief executive whenever he is in the air, was on a test flight a half-hour away. That was too long to wait.

Mrs. Kennedy was wheeled along an enclosed ramp into the hospital's sterile operating room. By that time, Dr. Walsh, assisted by four air force physicians, a military nurse, and five medics, was scrubbed in and awaiting her. Nearly careening through the operating room door, the medical staff made preparations for an emergency cesarean section. Soon, a blood transfusion would be necessary.

At Andrews Air Force Base, staff lined up a twin-engine, eight-passenger Lockheed JetStar, an aircraft lacking the equipment needed for in-flight communications and therefore never before used by the chief executive. As the plane taxied for takeoff at 12:30 P.M. to begin the 450-mile journey to Otis, the president sat alone. Seated near the president, Pamela Turnure recalled the moment:

> He was very withdrawn at that time. He just kept sitting and staring out of the window, and obviously his thoughts were completely with her. I had seen that look once before, when Jackie had gone into premature labor

with John Jr., and the President, who had just arrived in
Palm Beach, got the word, . . . "Come back."[48]

Patrick Bouvier Kennedy was delivered by cesarean section and
lifted head first from his mother's womb at 12:52 P.M.

His gestational age was thirty-four weeks. He measured seventeen
inches long from head to toe and weighed four pounds ten and a half
ounces. Yet he appeared well developed, with soft, light brown hair. Immediate movement of his tiny arms and legs was noted, as was his weak,
barely audible cry. Dr. Walsh assisted the newborn's initial respirations
using a suction device to clear his mouth and nasal passages of excess
secretions.

After the umbilical cord was clamped and cut, permanently separating mother from baby, the fragile infant was then handed over to Dr.
Walsh's assistant, who placed him in a waiting incubator.

At the time of Patrick's birth, immediate care for the newly born
was focused upon establishing respiration and conserving body temperature. For Patrick, this meant warmed blankets, a prewarmed incubator, the suction apparatus, and equipment for oxygen administration.

Yet, despite these stabilizing interventions, Patrick was unable to
establish a normalized breathing pattern. One of the doctors began in-
fusing oxygen into the incubator. Another repeated the suction procedure of both mouth and nose, aspirating little to nothing. Another
placed a stethoscope over Patrick's tiny chest, revealing shallow and
barely audible breath sounds. Maintaining the chart for the operation,
one physician wrote the infant's diagnosis: idiopathic respiratory distress
syndrome, translated as "difficulty in breathing for reasons unknown."

Infants who die from RDS, or associated complications, often display problems from their very first breath. That initial inhalation of air
for a baby at birth is his most important, and its successful execution is a
complex feat, containing much potential for hazard. The breath taken at
the moment of birth must expel the amniotic fluid contained within the

---

48. Nancy Tuckerman and Pamela Turnure, recorded interview by Mrs. Wayne
Fredericks, John F. Kennedy Library Oral History Program, 1964, 21.

lungs for them to fill with air. To accomplish this, the just-born infant must instantly generate ten to fifteen times more inspiratory pressure than she would normally.

The biological coordination that results in the infant's exchange of fluid for air must unfold in a flawless and well-timed sequence of events. During a normal vaginal delivery, the baby, descending the vaginal canal, has about a third of the fluid squeezed out of the lungs into the pharynx, where it oozes out of the mouth or is swallowed. Of the remaining fluid, about one-half is absorbed into the pulmonary capillaries, and half of that is absorbed into the pulmonary lymphatic system. The baby's vigorous cry signifies that the lungs have successfully made the conversion.

Patrick emitted no such cry. The staff in the operating room looked on anxiously as the infant's labored breathing indicated an inability to generate enough lung pressure to clear the amniotic fluid. Soon, his breathing rate escalated far beyond the normal newborn rate of forty to sixty breaths a minute. Rapid breathing is the baby's compensatory attempt to saturate the blood with as much oxygen as possible. An increased respiratory rate is one of five symptoms commonly associated with RDS and is termed *tachypnea*. Taking its name from the Greek *tachy*, meaning "swift," combined with *pnea*, "to breathe," tachypnea is observed as a rapid, shallow breathing rate, which in turn creates another distinctive symptom that the ancients referred to as *alae nasi flare*. Nowadays it is simply called "nasal flaring" and appears as an outward movement of the nostrils accompanying each inspiratory effort and signifying the infant's attempt to increase the diameter of his nasal airways to further increase airflow to the lungs.

Among the medical personnel surrounding the president's son, Patrick's rapid breathing and nasal flaring were recognized as precursors to RDS. Many of these professionals were devout Irish Catholics, and so they exercised the most logical and time-honored step: they called a priest.

8

The First Breath

And God breathed into his nostrils the breath
of life; and man became a living soul.
—Genesis 2:7, King James Version

Father John Scahill was the base chaplain and a Roman Catholic priest. When he appeared in the operating room to baptize Patrick, he was attired in the appropriate vestments for this highly ritualized act and carried a small bottle of holy water and a prayer book.

Placing his hands through the portholes of the incubator, he proceeded with the Latin rite of the Roman Catholic Church. While splashing the blessed water on the head, hands, feet, and arms of the infant, he recited the sacred benedictions that would formally admit Patrick into the Catholic faith. In reverence to the new life, Father Scahill said his invocations in a lowered voice, uttering prayers, devotions, and blessings. The emergency measure brought some comfort to the tension-filled staff even as it increased the fear for Patrick's fate.

Throughout the baptism, Patrick's breathing continued to accelerate. Anything that could help him had already been tried. There was nothing more to be done, and the medical staff responsible for his care stood helplessly by, mere observers who had to accept that they could only wait and pray that Patrick's tiny system would be blessed with the wherewithal to heal itself.

Throughout the baptism, Dr. Walsh remained quietly focused on Jackie. As he glanced over to Patrick's incubator, surrounded by anxious personnel, he was grateful that Jackie's deep sedation spared her the trauma of witnessing this scene, which might well be the start of her newborn's medical catastrophe.

Father Scahill spoke quietly and calmly about "God's will." The medical professionals had no patience for God's will and perhaps wondered why a loving God did not heal Patrick immediately. Their feeling would be echoed by the president in a few days, when his infant son was gone, his grief seemed insurmountable, and he wondered aloud why God would let a child die.

At 1:38 P.M., forty minutes after Patrick's birth, the president's jet descended onto the Otis airfield against the backdrop of a sunny Atlantic haze. JFK descended the stairwell of the small air force jet, where a waiting military police transport vehicle was waiting to rush him to Otis's hospital. Dr. Walsh had just completed his final sutures on Jackie's abdomen when the president arrived. The doctor at once informed the president that Mrs. Kennedy was fine but that the baby had breathing difficulties and required incubation with supplemental oxygen.

The president acknowledged his understanding of the situation while each, without mention, recalled John Jr.'s preterm birth accompanied by breathing difficulties and incubation treatment just three years before.

The fact that oxygen was being infused into Patrick's incubator indicated that the staff was treating another prominent symptom of RDS called *cyanosis*. From the Greek *cyan,* meaning "blue," and *osis,* "process of," the blue appearance of cyanosis indicates the failure of hemoglobin to carry enough oxygen to the tissues. Hemoglobin gives blood its bright red color, and when its contact with inspired oxygen is lost, the blood begins to take on a darker hue, a shade closely resembling the color of grape juice. Because the veins of the infant are the vessels closest to the surface, these thin-walled vessels, which cover the entire body, radiate the darkened coloring of the deoxygenated blood through the thin, nearly translucent skin, imparting a blue look to the skin that is particularly profound in Caucasian infants. Once known as blue baby syndrome, the blue discoloration is oftentimes related to infant cardiac disorders, though for the premature infant, the blue color is nearly always related to underdeveloped lungs.

9

The Infant Lung

There are two graces in breathing: drawing in air and
discharging it. The former constrains and the latter refreshes:
so marvelously is life mixed. Thank God then when he
presses you, and thank him again when he lets you go.
—Goethe (1749–1832)

If the Hubble Space Telescope could be turned inward to peer into an
infant's lungs, it would reveal a world that, like our universe, contains
its own cosmos and spatial relationships.

The human lung system is often referred to as the bronchial tree
because of its structural resemblance to an inverted tree. In the newborn, one could say the lung appears as a newly planted sapling. The
perception of the lungs as an inwardly growing tree also reflects the
biological fact that human lungs and trees share, as do all living organisms, both the physiologic basis of respiration and the goal of providing
oxygen. Whereas lungs provide oxygen to the inside of the human body,
trees, through photosynthesis, provide oxygen to the atmosphere, on
which humans, in turn, depend. If evidence is necessary to establish our
interdependence with the earth, there is no better proof than this.

Human lung buds appear in the fetus at the fourth week of embryonic development, thus beginning a process of constant motion that

continues throughout a human lifetime. Developing within a normal gestational period of thirty-seven to forty-two weeks, the newborn lung attains mechanical properties that give it the distinction of being the only internal organ to come in contact with the external environment.

At birth, each lung weighs about an ounce, or roughly thirty grams, and appears rounded and shaped similarly to a newly blossomed pear. When the lung fully develops into adult size, it appears more flattened and bell shaped, and the weight of each lung grows to a little over a pound, or about six hundred grams. Constructing themselves with a durability designed to carry their owner through a normal human life-span lasting some eighty years, the lungs' purpose is simple: to provide the body with oxygen and to remove carbon dioxide.

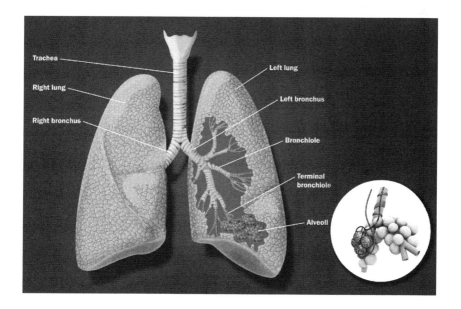

We normally do not think about the air we breathe, a remarkable fact when one considers that a healthy newborn breathes about seventy-two thousand times a day, while a healthy adult performs the task of breathing at least twenty-five thousand times each day. The adult human lung will convert thirty-two hundred gallons of air each day, transferring it as oxygen into the bloodstream.

Doctors, nurses, and respiratory care practitioners often think of air, referring to it simply as *room air,* which is the air that surrounds us in the atmosphere and contains as its primary constituents 21 percent oxygen and 78 percent nitrogen (the remaining 1 percent, known as trace gases, plays little, if any, physiologic role in respiration). When they discuss the merits of air to the infant and its consequences, they refer not to air in general but to a particular component of it: oxygen.

When Hippocrates stated that man was an "obligate aerobe," he was referring to the fact that without the intake of (oxygen-containing) air into and out of the lungs, the human species simply would not exist.[49] Even in his time, healers were aware that any interruption to oxygen delivery from our lungs to the rest of the body would result in death, though they did not know the reason for this.

The passage of air into newborn lungs follows a rather direct route, entering first through the nostrils of the infant. Known as obligatory nose breathers, infants breathe largely through their nares rather than through the mouth.

The vocal cords demarcate the upper airway from the lower airway, where the air actually enters the lungs. Traveling through the vocal cords, the airstream continues into and through the trachea, a small, tubelike structure measuring about five and a half centimeters in length and about the width of a drinking straw in diameter. The trachea is the largest part of the infant airway system. By comparison, the adult trachea is approximately twice as long and at least twice as wide.

As within the child and the adult, the infant trachea bifurcates into two distinct pathways, one leading into the right lung and the other into the left. These channels, called the right and left main-stem *bronchus,* from the Latin meaning "windpipe," immediately divide into three and two lobes, respectively. At each of these sites, the air continues its expedition, subdividing for another fifteen to seventeen divisional generations into ever narrowing branches. These tiny air passages then lead into what are fittingly called the *terminal bronchioles,* from the Latin

---

49. Oxygen was first isolated from the air in the eighteenth century, and the credit for coining the word goes to Antoine Lavoiser, who in 1777, initially termed it *oxygine.*

"ending airway passages," before finally entering into tiny microscopic air sacs called the *alveoli,* a term which, as previously mentioned, is derived from the Latin for "a small hollow or cavity." It is within the alveoli that the air finally comes to a halt and where nature's secret workroom can be found.

Similar in appearance to a balloon, the *alveoli* are highly elastic and permeable semispheres covered by two very thin layers of tissue. These are the single-celled capillary and alveolar walls. Their function is to separate oxygen from the air we breathe. The membranes separating this alveolar–capillary membrane are so thin as to be transparent, allowing minimal interference with the diffusion of oxygen into the blood and the diffusion of carbon dioxide out of it, a process known as *gas exchange.*

The lungs of the healthy, born-at-term infant each contain about 30 million alveoli, approximately 10 percent of the alveoli contained in a single adult lung. Seen microscopically, these tiny air sacs resemble bubbles suspended in a water solution. Because the micro-sized alveoli are not quite fully developed in the newborn lung, the surface area of the air sacs for gas (oxygen–carbon dioxide) exchange is only about 3 percent that in adult lungs, but this smallness is deceptive. If the total number of the infant's alveoli were spread out and flattened onto a level surface, the area they would cover would be about thirty-two square feet. The square footage is equivalent to the size of a typical office desk.

The alveoli continue to grow in number and size, a process termed alveolarization. When they are fully alveolarized at about two or three years of age, they will number an estimated 300 million per lung. Gradually, the square foot surface area of the alveoli continues to grow perhaps reaching maturity in the early teen years. By then, the cumulative size of the young adult air sacs is so large that if they were collapsed and the tissue spread out on a level surface, the surface area for gas exchange would be about the size of a racquetball court.

Surrounding the alveoli are capillary blood vessels that extract the oxygen from the alveoli by way of circulating blood molecules called *hemoglobin.* Enormous in size, hemoglobin makes up about 90 percent of the dry weight of each red blood cell and takes its name from the Latin *hem,* "blood," and *globis,* meaning "globe." Like metal slivers to a magnet, oxygen inside the alveoli binds with *hemoglobin,* which then converts into *oxyhemoglobin,* turning the color of blood to a bright red. Propelled by the heart's pumping action, the oxyhemoglobin is then circulated to the far reaches of the body's tissues, while simultaneously gathering up carbon dioxide, the body's waste product, and returning it to the lungs to be exhaled. Without too much effort, one can picture these huge globes being propelled around the infant body universe, picking up and dropping off their cargo.

Breathing also depends on a huge muscular organ called the diaphragm, which spans the width of the midsection and is connected on either side of the rib cage. Lying transverse directly below the lungs, the diaphragm is responsible for drawing air into and out of the lungs. As in the adult or child, exhalation occurs in the infant without exertion, allowing the diaphragm to return to its natural, billowed-up position. This natural recoil of the diaphragm and the elasticity of the lungs are facilitated by a thin layer of fluid coating the alveoli, called *surfactant.* Previously mentioned in chapter 2, surfactant is an abbreviated form of the words *surface active agent.* It allows the alveoli to expand during inspiration and to avoid their collapse when exhaling.

This is achieved when special cells in the alveoli produce surfactant, which appears as a foamy agent that functions as an elastic skin and envelops the alveoli, allowing for their expansion and contraction.

Surfactant not only sustains the elastic properties of the lungs, allowing for the lifetime ability to inhale and exhale, it also does such a good job of reducing the surface tension of the alveoli that the pressure within the well-developed and healthy infant lung is reduced to about seven to eight dynes (a dyne is a measure of force), allowing the alveoli to maintain their spherical shape throughout the human lifetime.

But in the absence of surfactant, the dyne in the baby's alveoli increases and the baby's lungs become stiff and rigid, leading to severe breathing difficulties and eventual collapse of the alveoli. The final chest X-ray of Patrick Kennedy's lungs would show signs of total alveolar collapse. The little boy's surface tension nearing the end of his life would be about thirty dynes, a figure associated with death by RDS.

At 2:10 P.M., Jackie, still groggy from sedation, was transferred from the operating room to her recovery room suite. While Secret Service agents stood in the vestibule outside the first lady's room, the president quietly entered. In the ensuing moments, they would be nothing more or less than a husband and wife who have had their difficulties and do not yet know they are on the verge of a tragedy that will transform their marriage and draw them closer than they have ever been.

It was not long before the president emerged from the room and went to get his first look at his newborn son. The incubator in which Patrick lay was surrounded by attending personnel. The small crowd immediately parted for the president and Dr. Walsh.

Patrick, with his tiny face and swatch of light brown hair, was a lovely baby, a baby breathing fast—very fast. A strange noise came from the incubator. The men drew nearer, and Dr. Walsh affirmed that the sound was coming from Patrick; it was an odd, high-pitched noise, a sound medical specialists refer to as grunting.

Originating from the same mechanism that allows a healthy baby to coo and cry, grunting is a phenomenon occurring when the glottis converts itself into a life-saving mechanism. The baby, in respiratory distress, holds the vocal cords closer together while exhaling forcefully against them, allowing air pressure to build inside the lungs. This creates pressure within the lungs that helps to support continued expansion of the alveoli. The increased pressure within the infant's lungs, when released against the nearly closed vocal cords, emits a tone so distinctive and music like that clinicians—rather than using the word *grunting*— refer to it as singing.

While JFK was becoming aware of his son's difficulties, his brother, Senator Edward (Ted) Kennedy of Massachusetts, was in Washington, D.C., presiding over the Senate. Suddenly, Majority Leader Mike Mansfield hurried into the Senate Chamber brandishing the press release announcing Patrick's birth. Senators of both parties rose and joined in a standing ovation, most of them aware that Patrick was the first child born to a sitting president since the birth of Grover Cleveland's daughter in 1893.

Within the hour, flowers and congratulatory messages poured in from religious leaders and political officials around the globe. The tone of these missives was the polar opposite of the gloom that had begun to descend over the hospital where Patrick lay in his incubator.

Patrick was just over an hour old. His breathing was ever more rapid and labored, requiring increasing amounts of oxygen. Though it was well known then that excessive oxygen could damage the eyes of the preterm infant, clinicians then, as they do now, provided oxygen as necessary to maintain adequate oxygenation to the baby. It is a delicate balancing act: too much oxygen could hurt the eyes, too little could damage the brain.

Dr. Walsh drew the president aside and told him that his son was afflicted with hyaline membrane disease. When making further references to the condition, he would have used the acronym that was standard then, HMD, though, as noted previously, the disease is known today as RDS.

Patrick's lungs were coated with a glassy membrane, the doctor explained. The goal was to keep him alive for the next forty-eight to seventy-two hours, which, the doctor said, should be long enough to allow Patrick to recover from the lung ailment.[50]

Walsh continued his conversation with the president. The odds of a positive outcome were fifty-fifty, but if Patrick survived the next few days, the likelihood was that he would recover with no lasting lung damage. In other words, the most important factor—and the only potential cure—was time itself. The matter at hand was how best to provide that

---

50. Dr. Will Cochran, an attending pediatrician at the Boston Lying-in Hospital in 1963, remarks, "When discussing with the parents the preterm baby with RDS, we would tell them that if they lived the first day, there was still a half a chance they would die, and if they lived the second day the odds of death would be 40 percent. If they survived the third day the odds of death would be reduced to 10 percent. If they passed the third day they almost always lived."

extra time. To that end, Kennedy instantly agreed with Walsh's suggestion to call Children's Hospital in Boston for a pediatric consultation.

Jim Hughes, chief resident in charge of inpatient services and new admissions at Boston Children's Hospital, answered Dr. Walsh's call.

To this day, Hughes recalls what followed in minute detail:

> The call came in as one of many that I would routinely receive throughout the day. I simply answered the page and the gentleman caller identified himself as Mrs. Kennedy's obstetrician [Dr. John Walsh] based in Washington, D.C. The caller explained that both he and she [Mrs. Kennedy] were currently up in Cape Cod where Mrs. Kennedy went into labor while vacationing. The caller proceeded to explain that Mrs. Kennedy's baby was born prematurely with breathing difficulties and he requested an immediate pediatric consult and transfer to Children's [Hospital]. . . . Following a short conversation in order to work out some details, the phone call then ended.

At first, Hughes wondered if the call was a hoax. He called his wife at home and asked her if it was true that Jackie was pregnant. When she said yes, Hughes realized the call was not a fake and instantly notified the admissions office and the chief of services to let them know that the hospital would be receiving a very special patient.

He then called Dr. James Drorbaugh, a composed forty-one-year-old instructor in the Department of Pediatrics at Harvard Medical School who Hughes knew as a highly respected pediatric physician and one very qualified to appreciate the special needs of premature babies.

When the call came, Dr. Drorbaugh was in his nearby office. Hughes presented the facts to him in a minimal amount of words. "The baby appears to be in significant respiratory distress. . . . Would you be willing to be the physician of record and go to see the baby and accompany his return to Children's [Hospital]?"

"Well," said Drorbaugh, "I've got a lot of patients in the office and I'm not sure if I can leave right away."

It occurred to Hughes that his request had not sunk in. "But the gravity of the call must have soon been realized," Hughes recalls with a wry laugh, "because he finally found a way for those patients to be taken care of so he could attend to the newborn son of the president of the United States."

Drorbaugh recounts the moments following Hughes's urgent phone call. "The first thing I did was take out the shoe shining kit I had in my desk drawer and shine my shoes. I think that was a reflex action to give myself a chance to adjust to what was going on. I then grabbed my doctor's bag and went outside and hailed a cab. We drove to the National Guard hangar at Logan Airport where I was met by air force staff. An aircraft had been prepared for takeoff and we immediately flew to the Otis Air Force Base hospital in Cape Cod."

Within an hour of Dr. Walsh's call, Drorbaugh arrived at the Otis Air Force Base. The president met him as he hurried off the aircraft, and the two men proceeded at a brisk pace to the Otis hospital while discussing Patrick's condition.

Upon seeing Patrick, Drorbaugh immediately noted that the infant was in significant respiratory distress. His physical condition appeared critical, prompting Drorbaugh to corroborate Dr. Walsh's suggestion that he be transferred immediately to Children's Hospital, a facility far better equipped to monitor and handle infants at risk.

While hospital officials prepared Patrick's emergency transport to Boston Children's, the president decided that, despite Patrick's condition, it was essential for Jackie to see her new child. The president and Dr. Drorbaugh walked behind Patrick's isolette as orderlies wheeled the incubator into the first lady's room. Inside the incubator, Patrick was breathing rapidly and was positioned so that he was facing his mother.

Dr. Drorbaugh was surprised to find Mrs. Kennedy fully alert mere hours after being anesthetized for her cesarean section. He edged the incubator closer to her and opened the porthole window. Gently she placed her hand inside it and stroked Patrick's light brown hair. But much-needed oxygen was escaping through the porthole, and her contact with her newborn son ended, of necessity, within mere minutes.

Dr. Drorbaugh then explained to her that Patrick had breathing difficulties and needed to be transferred to a place where he could be provided with advanced care. The president tried to soothe his wife's sense of alarm and profound apprehension, reminding her that John Jr. had had breathing problems too. Patrick, like John, would be better in a few days.

But it appears he didn't fully believe his own reassurances for, prior to leaving the hospital, he ordered that the TV set be removed from Jackie's room. Were Patrick to die, he did not want to imagine the possibility that she would hear of his death via television.

10

Patrick's Desperate Hours

We need men who can dream of things that
never were, and ask why not.
—epigraph contained in the White House diary the day
of Patrick's birth, Wednesday, August 7, 1963

At 5:50 P.M., Patrick was placed in an air force base ground ambulance to begin the sixty-mile journey to Boston. The motorcade was expedited by a police and military escort, and Dr. Drorbaugh, seated beside Patrick's incubator, was amazed to see armed law officers stationed on every overpass as well as Secret Service vehicles and motorcycle police clearing the way.

Dr. Walsh remained at Otis to attend to Jackie. At 6:18 P.M., the president flew from Otis to his Squaw Island vacation house to be with Caroline and John Jr. When the president sat down with his children to supper, he told them they had a new baby brother. He seemed to share in their excitement, though he made no mention of Patrick's condition.

Nearing 7:00 P.M., the ambulance arrived at the hospital, and Patrick's incubator was wheeled into a private room near the newborn nursery that had been hastily outfitted under Hughes's direction. Already gathered there to assess the infant were most of the senior staff at Children's Hospital and neonatal specialists from Boston Lying-in

Hospital. Dr. Wesley Boston, of the Boston Lying-in team, quickly and smoothly inserted an umbilical arterial catheter into Patrick's umbilicus to obtain a blood sample, which was then rushed across the street to Boston Lying-in, where there was a blood gas machine, one of few in existence nationwide.[51] This newly developed apparatus monitored acidic conditions of the blood as well as its oxygen and carbon dioxide contents. In time, it would prove so useful to clinicians seeking to guide infants to respiratory stability that it is today an essential component of NICU equipment.

The results of Patrick's blood gas analysis were soon reported, and as Drorbaugh suspected, the pO_2 (oxygen content of the blood) was down and the pCO_2 (carbon dioxide content of the blood) was elevated. To normalize Patrick's blood oxygen content, Drorbaugh added more oxygen to the incubator.

Shortly after eight o'clock, on the first night of Patrick's life, the president left his family's Squaw Island retreat and went, by helicopter, to the Otis hospital, where he spent half an hour with Jackie.

Departing Otis Airfield on Air Force One, he soon arrived at Boston's Logan Airport. There had been news reports of Patrick's breathing difficulties, and the cheering crowd that greeted him there seemed to be offering encouragement.

More people were waiting outside Boston Children's Hospital. The president offered a slight wave and attempted a smile as he hurried inside to be swiftly taken to the fifth floor, where he exchanged a few words with Dr. Drorbaugh.

Then, after donning a white gown and mask, he went into room 2534 to see Patrick.

Within, he could hear the quiet hum of the incubator and the steady beep of the cardiorespiratory monitor. Specialists, also wearing hospital gowns and masks, were gathered around the incubator, still evaluating the infant. The intravenous catheter remained in place for continuous fluid infusion, while a nearby oxygen tank, connected to the incubator via a flexible hose, provided a constant supply of gas.

---

51. Jim Drorbaugh, personal interview with the author, 2011.

Chest X-rays had been taken, and the latest of these revealed an increased hazy pattern in each lung, a typical RDS finding on the first day of life. Drorbaugh told the president there had been no change in Patrick's condition and that the infant's survival was still dependent on his body's ability to heal itself. The president's concern was palpable, but he remained collected and calm and was, as one of the doctors would later note, "very cooperative and knowledgeable, and picked up things very fast. He was a quick study."

One can only imagine how he felt; surely his feelings were those of any loving parent, but with a key difference: he was the most powerful man in the world, the only man in the United States who could order a nuclear strike, a man with armies at his command. Yet there he was, consigned to do nothing more than wait and hope and pray.

That sense of helplessness must have been compounded later that night, when he had retired to his family's apartment at the Ritz-Carlton. There, he read through the statement he planned to deliver to Congress about the Nuclear Test Ban Treaty, which he had negotiated with the Soviet Union and Great Britain, which banned nuclear testing in the atmosphere, in outer space, and under water.

As he read, it could not have been lost on him that, even as he made the world a safer place, he could not create a web of safety for his son.

11

Prayers for a Baby

Hope is the physician of each misery.
—Irish proverb

Dr. Drorbaugh sat beside Patrick's incubator throughout the night, in the room now guarded by Secret Service agents. Patrick's symptoms had not abated, and his accelerated breathing, nasal flaring, chest retractions, cyanosis, and severe grunting were nearing the outer limits of what his tiny body could support. The pediatrician couldn't think of anything worse than losing, on his watch, the son of the president of the United States, or anyone else's infant, for that matter. If he could only keep Patrick alive for another day or two, allowing time for the RDS to resolve on its own, there would be a chance for Patrick to recover.

At one point in the long night, Jim Hughes looked in on Patrick. He leaned over the incubator, unaware that his picture was being taken by a photographer from *Life* magazine, who had perched on an upper floor of a nearby building and was working with a telephoto lens. Nine days later, the black-and-white photograph picturing Hughes would appear on the cover of *Life,* over a headline that read, "Hospital Vigil Over the Kennedy Baby—Lighted Window A Compassionate Nation Watched."

Finally Thursday morning came, ushering in a warm summer day complete with tufts of clouds suspended against a luminous blue sky. In room 2534 of Boston's Children's Hospital, little Patrick seemed to be gathering strength, and his condition appeared stable.

By then, news of the infant's birth had been superseded by reports of his troubles, though the general belief, as stated in a *New York Times* editorial, was that "the initial infirmity is not considered serious."[52]

This editorial was titled "Prayers for a Baby" and captured precisely the widespread concern about Patrick's struggles:

> The world shares President Kennedy's vigil at the crib side of his new son. . . . In such moments of supreme personal trial, each of us is reminded of the irrelevancy of the daily tribulations that normally loom so monumental. . . . All Americans and countless others across the seas are united in prayer that the youngest of the Kennedys will soon be well.[53]

The president spent the morning going over his statement to Congress about the Nuclear Test Ban Treaty. It was without question a great achievement, a signature victory for history and for his administration, but as Kennedy read the triumphant statement aloud to his speech-writer, Ted Sorenson, there was only sorrow in his voice. More than any other persons in the world, Jack and Jackie Kennedy must have felt the poignancy of the strongest statement in that *New York Times* editorial: "What price the cold war, the posturings of General de Gaulle, the threat of a rail strike or slow motion in congress when measured against the value of this tiny life?"[54]

At 9:45 A.M., the president departed the Ritz-Carlton and motored to the hospital to confer with Dr. Drorbaugh, stopping first to see his son. When the doctor told him that Patrick's condition had stabilized, his first thought was to convey this welcome and somewhat unexpected news to Jackie.

---

52. Editorial, *New York Times*, August 8, 1963.
53. Ibid.
54. Ibid.

He boarded a helicopter at 10:17 A.M. and set off for the hospital at Otis Air Force Base. Maybe it really would be with Patrick as it had been with John Jr.: an alarming breathing crisis, followed by incubation, followed by robust health.

Jackie was buoyed by Patrick's improvement, so much so that she passed the afternoon picking out lipsticks in assorted colors and planning the entertainment for a state dinner to be held on October 1 in honor of Haile Selassie, the leader of Ethiopia and a man the president particularly admired. Jackie, a lifelong lover of dance, arranged for a ballet company to perform for the emperor.

Having promised Jackie that he would return at 4:00 P.M. for a brief visit before heading off to Boston to see Patrick again, Kennedy was helicoptered to the family home on Squaw Island, where Caroline and John Jr. were eagerly awaiting his arrival. Young John loved airplanes and was always thrilled and excited to see the helicopter with its twirling blades land on the lawn. The children raced to their father, who hugged them both but did not pick them up, for he had his own health issues, among them a bad back for which he had risked a surgery ten years earlier that would—he was assured—either greatly lessen his chronic pain or kill him.

By the time lunch was served on the terrace overlooking the water, they were joined by Jackie's mother, Janet Auchincloss, and her youngest daughter, also named Janet (Jackie's half-sister), then eighteen years old. Afterward, John Jr. dashed around the lawn on his sturdy little legs, bubbling over with joy and excitement. Sitting as parent and grandparent, JFK and Mrs. Auchincloss looked on, assured there was good reason to believe that, in the not-so-distant future, there would be two little boys on the lawn.

"He was always interested in what everybody in the world thought and felt . . . and honestly interested in how everybody reacted," said Mrs. Auchincloss in a 1964 interview.

> I will always remember what he said to Janet [Jackie's half sister] on the terrace outside of the house in

Hyannis Port on the day that I went to Boston with the President to see Patrick in the hospital where he had just been flown. When we were having lunch . . . Janet who was unhappy . . . who lacked self-confidence because she was a little bit overweight and self-conscious . . . was sitting outside on the grass, and Jack said to her, "You know, Janet, you're really a very beautiful girl." Her face lit up and she said, "Oh, Mr. President, I don't know what you mean." Just the fact that he said this to her gave her such a lift. . . . He was terribly understanding of young people.[55]   .

In the early afternoon, as John Jr. was scampering around, Patrick's breathing became more labored, and his blood gas measurement began to reflect increased clinical deterioration. Any hope of keeping him alive long enough for him to heal spontaneously was fading with a sudden and terrible swiftness. The doctors urgently conferred again.

"Bob Gross, chief of surgery at Children's, with senior staff came by to tell us that the hyperbaric chamber would be available if we thought we needed it," said Dr. Drorbaugh, recalling the moment. "Gross's offer was based upon his cardiac surgical team's experience using the chamber to operate on children with congenital heart disease."

The Children's Hospital pediatric staff, among the most accomplished pediatricians in the world, had done all they could to help Patrick, but the treatment was not working. All day long they had been flooded with calls from doctors from around the world offering clinical advice. These doctors would say, "Did you try this?" and "You should try that" or "You ought to do this." It was, thought Jim Hughes, a stunning influx of unsolicited input from everyone imaginable.

The course of action would rest with the hospital's senior staff, who reluctantly agreed there was only one treatment left to pursue: to move Patrick to a hyperbaric chamber, or "the tank," as it was often called,

---

55. Janet Lee Bouvier Auchincloss, recorded interview by Joan Braden, September 6, 1964, John F. Kennedy Library Oral History Program, pp. 24, 25.

in the hope that the infant would benefit from the pressurized oxygen within it.

Only one nearby doctor had considerable experience with the tank. He was Dr. William Bernhard, a Children's Hospital pediatric heart surgeon. An esteemed member of Dr. Bob Gross's cardiovascular team, Bernhard had discovered tremendous advantages utilizing the tank when operating on infants with certain cardiovascular disorders. By forcing super large amounts of oxygen into the babies, he had successfully performed more than a hundred operations inside the tank.

In the knowledge that Dr. Gross had made the hyperbaric available to the team, Dr. Drorbaugh phoned Dr. Bernard, who was in his laboratory when he received the phone call. Dr. Drorbaugh told him he had a newborn patient whose father was a member of an important family well known to the hospital's overseers.

They were doing everything they could to help him, Drorbaugh explained, but the baby was in severe respiratory distress.

"Would you come over and take a look at him?" Drorbaugh asked.

Bernard, in the moment unaware that the baby belonged to the president and first lady, replied, "I don't want any part of it."

"Ahhh," said Drorbaugh, "come over and have a look anyway."

Dr. Bernard headed over to the hospital, where he found a group of deeply concerned physicians gathered around Patrick's incubator, and where he discovered that the infant in distress was the son of the president of the United States.

Dr. Drorbaugh had another call to make, a tougher call, for this one was to Kennedy. The doctor spoke briefly and to the point, describing to the president how Patrick was taking a turn for the worse. Within minutes, the president and his mother-in-law had boarded the waiting helicopter and were on their way to Boston. The noise of the chopper's engines made conversation within the aircraft impossible. Perhaps the enforced silence was a welcome reprieve against emotions made unbearable, adjusting to the family crisis.

This baby is in rough shape, thought Dr. Bernhard. *He's working really hard to breathe.* Clearly even these exceptional doctors were having great difficulty stabilizing him. Now there was no way, he thought, that he could refuse to get involved. That settled, Dr. Drorbaugh explained why he'd summoned him: it had been decided by the hospital's senior staff to use the hyperbaric chamber to treat Patrick's RDS, although all involved were aware that the chamber had never been used to treat RDS.

Harvard's hyperbaric chamber, designed and built in 1928, was initially used by the navy for training submariners and decompressing divers and had not been used for more than thirty years when the innovative Dr. Bernhard began using it as an operating room for pediatric cardiac surgery.

The chamber operates on the theory that when air pressure is increased, oxygen dissolves more readily into the blood plasma and other physical solutions of the body. Carried throughout the body by circulation, this oxygen-enriched blood enters the body's tissues and saturates them with oxygen.

Ordinarily, Dr. Bernhard would not have put an RDS baby inside the hyperbaric chamber. But he was set on cooperating with these dedicated doctors. *They are trying so hard to save this baby,* he thought. *They feel they are losing the battle for his life, and want to try everything possible. This is a desperate and difficult situation and placement in the pressurized tank is a desperate measure.*

The helicopter bearing the president and Mrs. Auchincloss landed in a stadium near the hospital. Within minutes, Kennedy was at Patrick's side, and the doctors could see that, with one look at Patrick, he fully apprehended the gravity of the situation, for an infant in marked respiratory distress is an alarming and startling sight.

Often the baby lies on his back, with skin that has turned pale and gray. The hair is soft and shiny, with a downlike quality similar to a duckling's plumage and sometimes nearly as wet—a result of the humidity and temperature within the incubator, and the perspiration the baby creates breathing hard and fast over a sustained period. The effect is that the infant appears to have just stepped from a pond.

The legs are elongated and the palms of the hands and soles of the feet are extended upward. This classic posture, near prayerlike in comportment, evokes an attitude of transcendence, even as it suggests that the baby is preparing to surrender. The eyes are closed and the expression is akin to that of someone in a hypnotic state. The tiny head, often in a midline position, faces upward, nearly expressionless. This absolute stillness of the body is interrupted only by the movement of the nasal passages, which causes the nostrils to flare as respiration reaches a remarkable rate—often more than a hundred breaths a minute.

A conference was held in Patrick's room to discuss the latest developments. Two plans of action were agreed on. The first was an idea Patrick's grandmother, Mrs. Auchincloss, proposed, who insisted on bringing in for consultation Dr. Samuel Levine, a senior emeritus professor of pediatrics at Cornell University. The esteemed pediatrician had successfully managed the case of her other grandchild born premature, Anna Christina Radziwill, who was now three years old and doing well.

Then the doctors raised the possibility of placing Patrick inside the hyperbaric chamber. The hope was that the added pressure within the tank would force more oxygen into the tiny boy's bloodstream and buy enough time to allow the lung ailment to self-resolve. The doctors also discussed the risks, including blindness, from excess oxygen use. Senior staff members also explained to the president that this form of therapy had never been used to treat respiratory distress and would be a treatment of last resort.

Dr. Bernhard, in the course of discussions, told the president that it had to be clearly understood that the hyperbaric treatment would be a gamble.

The president was prepared to take that gamble. "Nothing must happen to Patrick," he told Mrs. Auchincloss, "because I just can't bear to think of the effect it might have on Jackie."[56]

Dr. Bernhard proceeded to gather his support personnel, who were proficient in the tank's usage. Soon the specialists were assembled beside

56. Janet Lee Bouvier Auchincloss, recorded interview by Joan Braden, September 6, 1964,
p. 25, John F. Kennedy Library Oral History Program.

the tank, which was located within the basement of the Shattuck Street building, a large gray stone medical building where Patrick was housed. Dressed in white smocks, technicians began checking out valves, wiring, compressors, motors, and the seals on the heavy iron chamber.

The white-enameled tank resembled a small submarine and measured thirty-one by eight feet. Attached to one side were a control booth and a two-way intercom.

As the tank was being readied, the recently retired Dr. Levine, personally phoned by the president, was picked up at his Manhattan apartment by New York City police. With sirens blaring, he was rushed (the wrong way down a one-way street) to the Butler aviation terminal at LaGuardia, where an air force JetStar was standing by to rush him to Boston.[57]

As his plane departed the New York airport, medical personnel began the transport of Patrick's incubator from the hospital to the basement of the adjacent Shattuck structure, where the hyperbaric chamber stood prepared and ready.

The air in that basement was pungent and musty. The massive iron tank resembled a wartime vehicle, and its odorous smell, its electrical components, and the lather of grease combined to create an atmosphere that seemed the antithesis of a healing environment, but it was Patrick's last chance.

57. Rachel Zimmerman, "Tale of the Pediatrician Snatched to Treat the Kennedy Baby," *CommonHealth Reform and Reality,* April 6, 2013, http://commonhealth.wbur. org/2013/08/tale-of-the-pediatrician-snatched-to-treat-kennedy-baby.

12

Patrick's Death

For of those to whom much is given, much is required.
—epigraph contained in White House calendar,
August 9, 1963, the day of Patrick's Death

It was 4:11 p.m., just over twenty-seven hours since Patrick's birth, when the incubator that contained him was carried into the hyperbaric chamber, followed by Dr. Drorbaugh, Dr. Bernhard, and Dr. Robert Smith, the chief of anesthesiology at Children's Hospital. The heavy doors were closed and locked tight. Beyond the tank's iron walls stood additional technicians and a small group of interns and senior staff physicians from Children's Hospital, among them Dr. Welton Gersony.

Dr. Gersony, then a first-year pediatric cardiology fellow, stood near his mentor, Dr. Alexander S. Nadas, a founder of pediatric cardiology. Nadas was also at the time highly knowledgeable of the effects of the hyperbaric chamber on babies with congenital heart disease.

According to Gersony, the president appeared fairly calm—as calm as one could expect of a parent with a sick baby.[58]

Dr. Nadas spoke to the president, explaining what the

---

58. Interview with the author, October 2014.

doctors were trying to do. The president repeatedly peppered Nadas with the question, "If Patrick survives, will he be mentally retarded?"[59]

The president was clearly thinking of his sister Rosemary, whose birth was interrupted by entrapment inside the birth canal, depriving her brain of oxygen and resulting in significant mental retardation. Nadas, known to be a huge Kennedy fan, sternly stated in his Hungarian accent, "Mr. President, we are trying to save the baby's life," after which President Kennedy abruptly stopped his inquiries.[60]

Dr. Gersony, who later became the Alexander S. Nadas Professor of Pediatric Cardiology at Columbia University and director of pediatric cardiology at Morgan Stanley Children's Hospital, continues:

> I was not involved in any clinical decisions regarding the baby's care. However, given that there was virtually no chance of survival, based on the profile of the laboratory findings, I share the view that it was reasonable to try the hyperbaric chamber. Just because it didn't work doesn't mean it was not worth the attempt. At that time, there were no effective treatments available to care for a premature baby in respiratory distress. When there are no standard options, and no hope, aggressive attempts are justified. New treatments can be discovered this way.[61]

Visually separated only by the tank's small porthole windows, the treatment teams communicated through a two-way intercom system. The console operator activated multiple electrical switches, and the

---

59. The relationship between mental retardation (now termed intellectual disability) and preterm birth then, as now, was considered a contributing factor to neurodevelopmental disabilities, chief among them cerebral palsy.
60. Ibid.
61. Ibid.

operating panel's colored lights came on. At first flickering, then glowing, the panel lights soon illuminated the gloom of the basement. The compressor motor started up, pumping while singing higher and higher until the sound settled into a sustained, high-pitched whir that echoed throughout the basement. While the tank was pressuring up with air, 100 percent oxygen was being fed directly into the incubator by means of a flexible hose connected to an external oxygen supply.

The normal atmospheric pressure exerted on a person is 14.7 pounds per square inch at sea level, which is measured as one atmosphere of pressure. The pressure inside Patrick's tank was set at three atmospheres, or 44.1 pounds per square inch—about three times the normal amount of pressure contained in the normal atmosphere. In addition, the oxygen content within Patrick's incubator was at 100 percent, about five times the amount taken in by a person living at sea level.

Inside the chamber's iron walls, Dr. Bernhard began monitoring readings in concert with the console operator, while Dr. Drorbaugh reassessed Patrick's condition. Drorbaugh, along with Dr. Bob Smith, eagerly watched the vertical spiked lines of the cardiorespiratory monitor attached by sensors to Patrick's chest, tracking and displaying both his heart and breathing rates.

During the time it took for the tank to reach maximum pressure, it seemed Patrick was responding favorably to the treatment. Within a few moments, doctors inside the hyperbaric saw an improvement in the EKG pattern.

It was at this hopeful time that Dr. Levine entered the basement and was guided to an observation area outside the hyperbaric chamber. There, hospital senior staff stood beside the president and Mrs. Auchincloss, who warmly greeted the elderly physician. Dr. Levine then recounted his incredibly fast journey from New York to the basement of the hospital. The retired Cornell University professor described how he had deplaned from the air force jet and been swiftly ushered into a waiting helicopter, which set down on a makeshift landing field at nearby Fenway Park. Levine continued, mentioning he was finally met by a Boston police cruiser that delivered him to the hospital with sirens blaring.

Dr. Levine told the president, "I'm very impressed with the efficiency of government!"

The president smiled. "It's about time you doctors learned that," he joked, clearly referring to the well-publicized debates regarding the American Medical Association's resistance to government intervention.

Dr. Levine was surprised to find that Patrick was in the oxygen chamber and was perturbed that, because of this, he could not examine him. With Patrick inside the tank, which rendered him helpless to perform a physical assessment, he instead perused the baby's chart and studied the X-rays. For more than thirty minutes, he discussed Patrick's condition with doctors intimate with the case. All were unanimous that the young Kennedy had proceeded into an advanced stage of respiratory distress and that there was no way to treat the cause from which the symptoms originated.

Like every other doctor on Patrick's case, Dr. Levine was forced to accept that the infant's sole chance of survival depended on the intervention and success of the hyperbaric tank.

In the late afternoon, the president returned to the Ritz-Carlton. After some time alone, he called his secretary, Evelyn Lincoln, who had set up a temporary office in the hotel. He asked her to bring him some personal stationery. When she entered his room, she found the president seated on the bed, staring into space.

She thought, *This man is really suffering.* She waited in the doorway for a full minute before he became aware of her presence. As she handed the stationery to him, she asked, "How are things with little Patrick?"

"He has a fifty-fifty chance."

"That's all a Kennedy needs," she said. "He will make it."[62]

The president did not respond to her words of encouragement. Instead, he asked her to wait while he wrote a note. "Please find enclosed a contribution to the O'Leary fund. I hope it is a success."[63] The O'Leary Fund had been set up to benefit the family of James O'Leary, a Boston policeman killed while performing his duties. Kennedy placed in an

---

62. Lincoln, *My Twelve Years with John F. Kennedy,* 294–95.
63. Ibid., 296.

envelope both the note and a check for $250, an amount approximating $1,800 in today's currency. He told Mrs. Lincoln to give the envelope to one of the Secret Service agents to deliver.

He was so distressed that, some time later, when the check was presented at the bank, Mrs. Lincoln would receive a call from a bank officer seeking to ascertain whether the indecipherable and unfamiliar signature on it was really that of President Kennedy.

The time was nearing eight o'clock on Thursday night. Patrick was nearing thirty hours old.

Deep inside the basement of the Shattuck Street building, more than three hours had passed since the infant had been placed inside the tank. The president had resumed his watch in the basement, joined in the vigil by the two men who were closest to him: his brother, Attorney General Robert Kennedy, and Dave Powers, a special assistant to the president who had been with JFK since his first campaign—for a congressional seat—in 1946.

As the tank hissed and clanked and the high-speed compressor whined, technicians standing outside the hyperbaric tank kept watch over the internal pressure, making sure it maintained three atmospheres.

Inside the tank, Dr. Drorbaugh, Dr. Smith, and Dr. Bernhard closely monitored Patrick, their feelings alternating between hope and doubt. The grim, bluish skin color had returned; the infant's struggle to breathe was intensifying. Would the hyperbaric treatment be enough to carry Patrick through this crisis period and to a point where his body's natural repair system would help resolve his respiratory distress? As the doctors looked on at the side of their tiny patient, their initial optimism over his apparent progress descended into uncertainty, which quickly progressed to grave doubt.

At 8:30 P.M., the doctors met with the president. Dr. Bernhard quietly told him, "I think we're not going to be able to provide help for the little boy."

While the stricken father struggled to take this in, the doctor added, "If we have to insert a breathing tube into the infant's trachea and ventilate with a hundred percent oxygen that would indicate further deterioration."

Dr. Bernard had not voted for Kennedy, but he was aware that they had some things in common: both had served as naval officers in World War II, and both were parents. Like every doctor on the case, Bernhard was deeply impressed by the president's cooperative nature, his knowledge, and his steadiness in the face of the worst crisis a parent can face. Bernhard was not a man given to sentimentality, but it struck him that Kennedy was, as he would note later, "a wonderful father."

The president and Bobby Kennedy remained outside the tank while the Secret Service and hospital administrators sequestered the doctor's lounge on the fourth floor of the adjacent Farley Building and moved in a bed and television set for the president. Sometime after that, the two Kennedys and Powers went to the fourth-floor lounge to await the next medical conference at 11:00 P.M. The president was silent, restless, and distraught. Time passed with agonizing slowness. Finally it was time to return to the basement for the scheduled conference.

While they waited for an elevator, the president paced the corridor, walking down and back until he noticed, in one of the glassed-off rooms, a small child who had been severely burned.

He approached the nurse on duty and asked how the accident had happened. Then he asked, "Does the child's mother visit often?"

"Every day," the nurse said.

"Would you tell me her name?" Kennedy asked.[64]

The nurse complied. Then Kennedy asked Powers for a pen and a piece of paper. On it, above his signature, he wrote, "Keep up your courage."[65]

In those four words he told her what he must have been telling himself.

The doctors told the president that Patrick's condition was worsening.

Dr. Bernhard recalls, "He was not going to last long unless we put a tube in. Back then you would almost never start out intubating a

---

64. O'Donnel and Powers, *"Johnny, We Hardly Knew Ye,"* 428–29.

65. Clarke, *JFK's Last One Hundred Days.* 17.

baby unless they were struggling and death was imminent and no other choice was available. Intubation was a last resort, and you could almost be assured you were going to lose a baby when it got to that point."

At about 7: 00 P.M., according to Drorbaugh, just after Patrick had experienced a prolonged apneic (without breathing) spell, Dr. Robert Smith slipped a small breathing tube into the infant's tiny lungs. He then began ventilating, or "bagging," the baby using a small, handheld lung inflation device called an ambu bag, which is a rubber apparatus about the size and shape of a small football. The action was designed to help Patrick maintain proper pressure inside the lungs. The device made a whooshing sound within the tank's cramped quarters.

Watching and listening, Dr. Bernhard thought, *Things are slipping away.*

At this point, Patrick appeared to be in less respiratory distress for the very reason that he was becoming less able to summon the energy and effort required to breathe rapidly. Like a boxer who cannot go one more round, the RDS infant becomes fatigued from breathing so quickly and for so long and begins to wear out.

The president was urged to get some rest. He agreed to try but insisted on remaining as close as possible to Patrick. Rather than return to the fourth-floor lounge, he determined to spend the night in the basement boiler room adjacent to the tank, where a couch was hastily placed. Kennedy sat down on the couch. He was not ready for sleep.

The steady noise emanating from the massive chamber echoed throughout the basement and combined with the hissing of pressurized gas and the clanging sound of metal against metal. The president rose repeatedly and went across the hall where he looked in through the porthole at the solemn doctors still attending his son. It was well after midnight when he removed his jacket, loosened his tie, and took off his shoes. Before lying down, he dropped to his knees and prayed, as he had every night of his life.

While Thursday night slipped into Friday morning, inside the hyperbaric chamber, staff members—still hoping for a miracle—began to prepare themselves for the end. Patrick's diaphragm was pumping with such force that the collapsed lung tissue had begun to stretch and tear, increasing the inflammatory process.

Because his lungs had been failing in their job, his heart, to compensate, was beginning to wear out from beating so quickly against increasingly stiff lungs. It was, for any doctor well acquainted with RDS, a familiar and terrible sequence: the heart begins to fail, reducing its output of blood, in turn causing circulation to back up, which results in dangerously high amounts of fluid accumulating in the lungs. This fluid buildup is referred to as pulmonary edema, a term derived from the Greek *pulm*, meaning "lung," and *oidema*, "swelling."

One of the more striking features of severe infant RDS is the depth and force of each spontaneous breath. Each desperate heave of the infant diaphragm is an attempt to draw in air, while severe carbon dioxide retention increases. This breathing pattern indicates a far greater degree of collapsed alveoli, or atelectasis, forcing the baby to breathe even harder in a vain attempt to reinflate collapsed air sacs. A comparison can be made to blowing up a child's balloon, which becomes easier to do as the balloon becomes more inflated. However, once the balloon begins to deflate, the effort to keep the balloon inflated becomes that much harder.

The doctors seated beside Patrick observing the classic breathing pattern could do nothing other than manually inflate the lungs and watch him suffocate to death.

At 2:10 A.M., one of the Secret Service agents roused Dave Powers, who was sleeping near the president in the basement room, and told him that Patrick's condition was taking a bad turn. The president then felt Dave's hand on his shoulder, shaking him gently awake.

Kennedy walked quickly back to the tank only to encounter the voice of Bill Bernhard speaking through the intercom. It had fallen to him to do the most difficult thing a man of medicine has to do. "We are losing," he told Kennedy.

It's important, thought Bernhard, *that he is prepared.*

The president sat silently beside the tank, on a simple wooden chair. Within the tank, Patrick lay on his back.

His tiny arms and legs were losing muscle tone and taking on a floppy appearance, an indication that his oxygen-deprived brain was no longer able to send signals to contract his muscles.

Patrick's spontaneous breathing rate lowered to fewer than twenty breaths a minute, signaling that his diaphragm and lungs were failing to function. At the same time, each breath became less labored and more shallow. The baby's breathing finally quieted and he became more peaceful, while the anesticist continued manually inflating the baby's lungs.

Patrick's oxygen-starved brain allowed for rapid cellular death, which rendered his nervous system incapable of regulating itself. His heart rate began to descend from a fixed pattern well past a hundred beats per minute to a rhythm of far fewer that number. These last two findings are particularly ominous and signal impending death.

As the hour approached 4:00 A.M., JFK stood beside the tank, separated from his dying son by the steel walls. There were tears in his eyes. Inside the chamber, obscured from his view, powerful floodlights illuminated Patrick inside his isolette. The intercom became silent. Each of Patrick's inspirations had become a violent gasp. These concluding breaths are termed the *agonal phase* of breathing, from the Greek *agon,* meaning "struggle." The infant's breathing rate descends to fewer than fifteen breaths a minute, then drops to ten, beginning a rapid decrease to what is referred to as *apnea,* from the Greek "without breathing."

Following complete apnea, the heart of an infant or toddler continues to beat for a short while. It then begins its final descent. This descent continues, sometimes for just another few minutes, and sometimes longer.

Patrick's heart beat for the last time at 4:04 A.M.

He was thirty-nine hours old.

Kennedy was standing with his brothers, Bobby and Ted, and Dave Powers when word came through the intercom that it was over.

Kennedy walked away, seeking the privacy of the hospital's boiler room. There he wept for ten minutes.

When he returned, Bobby put an arm around his shoulders.

Quietly, the president said, "He put up quite a fight. He was a beautiful baby."[66]

Drorbaugh recalls the moment. "After Patrick died we had to wait inside the chamber for several hours while it decompressed before we could come out. The Children's Hospital staff who had been with us when we went into the chamber stayed to support us and met us when we came out. The president was not there.

Drorbaugh continued, "We shared our feelings of sadness with the senior staff and then we went our separate ways. My home was within walking distance of Children's Hospital so I walked home. It was daylight by then."

The president was still weeping when he left the hospital and set off for Otis Air Force Base, where Jackie awaited him. His expression was bleak and his eyes were red when he entered her room, where the bereaved parents wept together.

Later that morning, the president phoned Dr. Drorbaugh, who remembers that call with a special clarity. "He thanked me for trying to help his son. I told him how sorry we all were that we had not been able to help. He said he thought it just was not in the cards."

A few weeks later, Drorbaugh and the other doctors received a small framed portrait of the White House personally inscribed by the first lady: "For Dr. James Drorbaugh with deep appreciation."

"A very tragic episode was made more bearable," says Drorbaugh, "because of their graciousness towards all of us every step of the way."

Mrs. Kennedy, still recuperating from her C-section, was too frail to go to the funeral Mass, which was held the day after Patrick died. Attending were the president, his two brothers and their wives, Mrs. Auchincloss, and a handful of other close family members. Cardinal "Richard James" Cushing presided over the proceedings, which were held in his private chapel.

While the president stood alone weeping in the first pew, the cardinal recited the Mass of the Holy Angels, a Roman Catholic service for the infant dead.

As the service ended, Kennedy reached into his pocket and withdrew a gold Saint Christopher medal fashioned into a money clip which had been given to him by Jackie as a wedding present. Saint Christopher is the patron saint of travels and travelers, and the medallion is associated with safekeeping while traveling; since the day of his wedding, it had been a constant possession inside the president's pocket. Now, as Patrick was set forth on his final journey, Kennedy placed the medal in his son's tiny white coffin.

Following the ceremony, the other mourners left the chapel and began the ten-minute drive to the Kennedy family burial plot at Brookline's Holyhood Cemetery near the president's birthplace. Kennedy stayed behind, so overwhelmed with grief that he put his arm around the casket and held it tight.[67] To the cardinal, it looked as if he would never let go.

"Come on, Jack," the Cardinal said. "Let's go. God is good."[68]

At the cemetery, the coffin was placed in the ground, as the president wept.

The Pathophysiology of RDS

The branch of medicinal study dealing with the cause and effect of disease is called *pathophysiology.* Taking its name from the Greek prefix *path,* connoting a "condition of suffering," and *physis,* meaning "nature," combined with *logos,* or "reason," the term poetically defines the study of disease as the "reason behind nature's suffering."

Like many other preterm babies of the time who died by RDS, Patrick was asphyxiated by his lungs' inability to produce surfactant, the liquid film that coats the inside of the lungs.

Acting as an elastic skin allowing for the lung to expand and contract, *without collapsing,* special cells responsible for producing surfactant appear as early as the twenty-week gestational period. The cells generally delay full production of surfactant until about the thirty-fifth week of

---

67. Richard Cardinal Cushing, recorded interview by Edward M. Kennedy, John F. Kennedy Oral History Program, Boston, MA, 1966, 18.

68. Ibid.

gestation, and for this reason, most babies born after that time do not show signs of respiratory distress.

When preterm infants are born deficient in surfactant, this appears to rig the first of two stages allowing for the formation of the *hyaline membranes* inside the infant alveoli.

The first phase begins when the surfactant-deficient alveoli rob the lungs of their ability to expand and contract, causing their collapse, a function not unlike a child's balloon losing its air. The collapsed alveoli, in turn, decrease the amount of oxygen available to enter the bloodstream. This in turn causes the capillary blood vessels, which envelop the alveoli, to narrow, eventually obstructing the blood supply to both the alveoli and their tiny air passages (bronchioles). This sequence of events permits the cells within the lung tissue to die.

In the second phase, the dead cells ooze their way into the air sacs, while plasma (the liquid part of the blood, composed of 92 percent water and 7 percent protein) begins to leak from the capillary blood vessels into the alveoli. The combination of the dead cellular debris and plasma fills the alveoli, thus forming the hyaline membrane, a barrier that interferes with the penetration of inhaled air into the lungs. Once the hemolytic ooze fills the alveoli and its penetration is complete, lack of aeration occurs. The result is that oxygen cannot be taken into the bloodstream, and carbon dioxide cannot escape to be exhaled out.

As an illustration of how the hyaline membranes form, we can return to the bronchial tree—or sapling—as an analogy. Let's now imagine that the young tree is hollow and that its trunk (trachea) feeds into the branches (primary airways), leading into the twigs (generational airways), leading finally into the leaves (alveoli). Envision then the entire inside of the hollow tree, the trunk, the branches and twigs, leading into the leaves, all becoming progressively narrower, eventually closing off to the point where they begin to suffocate for lack of air and nutrients, resulting in a thick, clear sap that coats the inside of the leaves (the hyaline membrane). The tree, in essence, strangles itself.

13

Hope for the Newborn at Risk

Hope is a Waking Dream.
—Aristotle (fourth century B.C.)

The death of Patrick Bouvier Kennedy stunned the nation, but it also placed a world spotlight on a lung ailment that had been killing tens of thousands of babies each year.

Although the menace of RDS was well known to the medical community during the time leading up to Patrick's death, only a small group of scientists were dedicated to finding a treatment, all of whom were deeply impacted by Patrick's death. Those laboring inside Jeremiah Mead's Harvard lab, including Mary Ellen Avery, became more determined than ever to find a way to treat RDS.

Following centuries of agonizingly slow evolution of newborn care, Patrick's death began to arouse very deep and public-spirited forces.

Just two days following Patrick's death, Pierre Salinger, the White House press secretary, received a personal letter from Alfred Benesch, a Cleveland attorney who had been deeply shaken by Patrick's death. He wrote that he and his fellow Harvard alumni supported the "establishment of a fund for the study of the ailment that caused the tragic death of Patrick Bouvier Kennedy."[69]

---

69. Alfred A. Benesch to Pierre Salinger, August 9, 1963, White House Central Subject Files, box 709, John F. Kennedy Library, Boston, MA.

Salinger, also profoundly hurt by Patrick's death, in turn sent a letter to Jim Drorbaugh. His letter appears to be the first documented exchange about funding for newborn RDS between a ranking Kennedy administration official and the doctors who had cared for Patrick. Salinger wrote,

> Dear Dr. Drorbaugh,
> I am enclosing a copy of a letter received by a Cleveland attorney. I would appreciate your views on the proposal.[70]

Recently, Dr. Drorbaugh and I discussed his response to the letter Salinger wrote to him fifty years ago. He said, "Salinger's letter requesting input about setting up a special fund for HMD [now RDS] was received at a time when many of us in the newborn medical community felt frustration at not being able to do more for Patrick or any of the newborns with HMD. So when he personally asked me about setting up a government-sponsored fund it sure seemed like a great opportunity to get significant funding for neonatal research benefiting every aspect of newborn care, especially RDS."

In a letter dated August 29, 1963, Dr. Drorbaugh responded to Salinger's request:

> Dear Mr. Salinger,
> . . . The proposal of a fund for the study of Hyaline Membrane Disease sounds like a good one to me. . . . However, I do not know of any foundation that is exclusively interested in the problems of the newborn. . . . I think the fund should be thought of as a "fund for the furthering of neonatal research since the problems of hyaline membrane disease are really the problems of a newborn premature infant."
> Sincerely yours,
> James E. Drorbaugh[71]

---

70. Pierre Salinger to James E. Drorbaugh, August 22, 1963, White House Central Subject Files, box 709, John F. Kennedy Library, Boston, MA.
71. James E. Drorbaugh to Pierre Salinger, August 29, 1963, White House Central Subject Files, box 709, John F. Kennedy Library, Boston, MA

Although I found no evidence that Salinger had communicated Drorbaugh's views to the president on the RDS matter, the fact that the president and Salinger were near-constant companions gives little reason to doubt that the topic was not thoroughly discussed between them.

In any case, what soon came to pass in those sorrow-filled days would predetermine the course of newborn care for decades to come.

Eunice Shriver, the president's sister who helped him establish the National Institute of Child Health and Human Development (NIHCD) just one year earlier in October of 1962, recalls the mournful period following Patrick's death.[72] Addressing the president's concerns regarding proposed NIHCD programs and diseases of the newborn, Shriver recalls being questioned:

> He was interested in children's diseases . . . and he had a rather sympathetic outlook on children. I remember out on the boat once he said to me why did he have to support another institute . . . because it was going to cost a lot more money and he was having trouble with the budget and . . . I told him about virtually nobody studying anything about infant mortality or with very little knowledge about prenatal diseases and that sort of thing. And I said, "What about your own son? You probably wouldn't have lost one of your children if we knew more about prematurity." He said, "Are they going to study that kind of thing at the NIHCD, prematurity and that sort of thing?" I said, "Yes, Jack. And then that's what's going to stop it." And he said, "Well, that seems to really be worthwhile."[73]

Fewer than eight weeks later, on the crisp, chilly morning of October 24, 1963, a light rain fell on the great landscape of the White

---

72. Eunice Kennedy Shriver, recorded interview by John Steward, May 7, 1968, pp. 26, 27, John F. Kennedy Library Oral History Program.
73. Ibid., 26.

House grounds. Inside, in the cabinet room, members of the press were readying themselves for a major news conference. At 11:30, the president approached the podium and in the next few minutes signaled what would be a seismic shift in American child and newborn care:

> Ladies and gentlemen: it gives me great pleasure to approve this bill . . . which strengthens our maternal, and child health and crippled children's services. . . . Studies indicate infants born prematurely are ten times more likely to be mentally retarded. Mothers who have not received adequate prenatal care are two to three times more likely to give birth to premature babies. . . . This bill will help insure that no child need be born retarded for such reasons, which are wholly in our control.

The president then signed into law a massive grant authorizing a $265 million (nearly $2.1 billion in today's dollars) expenditure over five years, a large portion to be used for newborn research. Sponsored by the NIHCD, the bill was titled the Maternal and Child Health and Mental Retardation Planning Amendments of 1963.

The president continued to be concerned with the status of research on RDS, sending a series of memos requesting hyaline membrane disease, or RDS, updates to presidential science advisor Dr. Jeremy Weisner. In a letter dated November 6, 1963, just days before the president's death, Weisner responded to the president's inquiry:

> You inquired recently about the status of research on HMD which, as you know, is included in the program of NIH in the area of Child Health and Human Development. We have had a discussion with the institute director, Dr. Robert Aldrich, and are able to report that the entire program is developing very well with respect to organization, research plans, and recruitment of personnel. . . . At the present time NIH is funding a total

of $1,283,000 for grants to study premature onset of labor. Of this sum $800,000 [$6.2 million in today's dollars] (44 grants) is devoted specifically to hyaline membrane disease. . . . You will also be interested in the attached tabulation of infant mortality in various countries. It emphasizes better than anything else the necessity of a vigorous program in the fields of parental and child health. . . . You will note that between 1950 and 1962 the United States tumbled from 6th to 11th place in the ranking.[74]

The massive infusions of grant money would marshal scientific resources to support fetal lung research and find a way to treat RDS.

Only five years later, in 1968, Emile M. Scarpelli, a professor of pediatrics and physiology at the Albert Einstein College of Medicine, would write the first scholarly, detailed study on the subject of pulmonary surfactant, titled *The Surfactant System of the Lung*.[75] He listed nearly 330 references to research papers on infant lung research disease. Well over 250 of those studies were undertaken following Patrick's death. The fact is significant when considering the amount of time necessary for research to reach the printed page.

Because Patrick's death had also brought focus to the necessity of improved neonatal care for preterm and other high-risk neonates, the ensuing decades saw the proliferation of NICUs designed and built specifically for the special needs of newborns at risk.

Manufacturers in the decade would also respond to the issue of infant RDS by designing ventilators and associated equipment especially tailored to meet the infant's needs. Among other developments, this would lead to the introduction of the now famous "baby bird" ventilator in 1971, the first mass-produced breathing machine tailored for newborn support.

---

74. Jerome B. Weisner, MD, John F. Kennedy Presidential Library and Museum, Office of Science and Technology, Digital Identifier JFKPOF-085-011, November 6, 1963, Columbia Point, Boston, MA.
75. Scarpelli, *Surfactant System of the Lung*.

The search for a pharmaceutical therapy to treat RDS would lead, in 1990, to the development of the first synthetic pulmonary surfactant drug, Exosurf, approved by the U.S. Food and Drug Administration for newborn care. Considered by many to be the holy grail of pharmaceutical treatments for RDS, the drug, milk-like in consistency, is squirted directly, via a breathing tube, into infant lungs, most often resulting in near-instantaneous improvement. In fact, surfactant therapy, remarkable in its prompt effect, would also have a near-immediate effect on nationwide infant death rates. It is significant that "eighty percent of the decline in the U.S. infant mortality rate between 1989 and 1990 could be attributed solely to the use of surfactant."[76] So revolutionary was this therapy that it divided the world of infant medicine into what are now known as the pre- and postsurfactant eras, the time before 1990 and the years following.

Forty-nine years after Patrick's death, in 2012, the NICHD would list its accomplishments since becoming operative in 1963 during the Kennedy administration.[77] The most significant of these accomplishments was that "survival rates for respiratory distress syndrome have gone from 5% in the 1960s, to 95% today, due to advances in respirator technologies and the availability of replacement lung surfactant."[78] Today, RDS is one of the most treatable diseases among newborns as well as the most curable. In other words, had Patrick Bouvier Kennedy been born today, his survival would have been virtually assured.

The huge advances in neonatal care do not mean that the formerly compromised infant is now entirely safe from the corporeal realities of being born too soon. At the time of this writing, one out of eight infants born in the United States is born premature—twice the number of 1963, when premature births occurred in one of every sixteen infants. Among the many elusive factors affecting this high rate of prematurity

76. Schwartz et al., "Effect of Surfactant on Morbidity, Mortality, and Resource Use in Newborn Infants."
77. http://www.nih.gov/about/almanac/historical/legislative_chronology.htm#nineteensixty.
78. http://www.nichd.nih.gov/about/overview/mission/Pages/index.aspx

is the increased population of mothers who are obese, hypertensive, and diabetic and, in many cases, living below the poverty line. Additionally, smoking, poor nutrition, and drug and alcohol use remain contributing factors.

Also implicated as a cause of preterm birth over the last several years are women thirty-five years and older, euphemistically called advanced maternal age, who delay marriage and childbearing. That suggests that an older maternal age is a risk factor for premature birth. Associated with the trend to delay childbearing is the dramatic rise in the use of fertility treatments in the last twenty years. Among those pregnancies conceived through assisted fertilization, more than half result in multiple births. In that population, 62 percent of twins and 97 percent of triplets are born premature.[79] Notably, assisted in vitro fertilization (IVF) procedures that result in a single baby conceived are twice as likely to end in preterm birth.[80]

All of the described conditions share the common thread of being preventable. Now, as in Patrick's time, the preterm population remains at risk for developing RDS. But what that portends for the mortality of these infants has totally changed. Nowadays, most infants following a standard course of RDS in the NICU are routinely treated and discharged home. Finally, the long and slow evolution of the care of the newborn has found its formula and permanent ground on which to stand.

Laura's Story

Among the millions of babies who have benefited from newborn medical advancements since Patrick's time is a young woman I will call Laura, born in the presurfactant year of 1980. Born weighing only two pounds one ounce at a gestational age of twenty-eight weeks, I first met her as a teenage hospital volunteer in the very same NICU where I practiced and where she had spent the first three months of her life. Now a thirty-four-year-old registered nurse, her experience as a premature infant led to her decision to attend nursing school. She is now

---

79. Behrman and Stith Butler, *Preterm Birth*, 16, 17.
80. Ibid.

an NICU nurse, a living example of precious hope to parents she meets in the NICU. Though I was not involved in her care, several of my older colleagues were. They confirmed she was connected to the ventilator for at least three months. She was kept alive thanks to the "baby bird" breathing machine and other equipment newly tailored for newborn use. Today, she is a healthy and radiant woman with no signs of her death-defying transformation.

Sharing some details of the episode, Laura says, "My lungs were very underdeveloped and stiff from lack of surfactant. I was on the ventilator for a long time and had no less than four chest tubes in place [placed due to air leaks in the lungs]. The doctor told my mom and dad my chances for survival were at most 20 percent."

She said the doctors had also told her parents that the chances of her incurring cerebral palsy and other neurologic deficits were high, a consequence not uncommon for extremely premature infants.

"In high school I received mostly As and Bs, and graduated near the top of my class in nursing school."

Nowadays, because of the development of lung surfactant, it's likely Laura would not have had chest tubes or been connected to the ventilator for such a long period of time, which brings me to tell Missy's story.

Missy's Story

Another young woman I know, whom I will call Missy, was born in the postsurfactant year of 1995. With a birth weight of only one pound eleven ounces, she was born at twenty-nine weeks' gestation. Once again, I did not have far to look to find her or her mother, whom I will call Janet, a current colleague and a highly skilled neonatal nurse who was inspired to attend nursing school after Missy's birth. "When I was pregnant with Missy," she says,

I was consigned to seven weeks of bed rest and so what I remember most about her birth is the relief I felt when she was born. She was born in the wee hours of the morning and the room filled with harried medical personnel who took her away before I knew what happened. I was only sixteen years old and had no idea what a newborn intensive care area was, but soon found out. When I first saw her a few hours after birth, she was so tiny though breathing comfortably thanks to nasal continuous positive airway pressure, a mild form of respiratory support.

I was told that she had received surfactant for her serious RDS which immediately stabilized her breathing pattern. Despite a couple of scares that did not have anything to do with her breathing she was discharged from the hospital nine weeks later, a time approximating her original due date. When I brought her home, she weighed five and a half pounds.

Remarkably, Missy is also an occasional volunteer in our NICU. Now in her senior year in high school, she is a teenager whose picture could be found in a teen magazine. Healthy and intelligent, she is "chatty" and loves swimming, playing tennis, and participating in school activities. Although not yet sure what she wants to do following high school, she says nursing school is definitely "on the map."

Nowadays, the vast majority of preterm births follow a routine course of treatment, like that of Missy, and like Missy, most preterm babies will be discharged to home at the approximate time of their original due date.

Although it cannot be stated that the death of Patrick Kennedy on August 9, 1963, was the sole event that changed the course of newborn medicine, no one can dispute that it took the death of the president and Jackie's baby to bring RDS and the infant mortality rate into modern public focus.

The progress in infant research that sprang from that event and time excelled with a pace that may have no equal in the history of scientific medicine. Since the early 1960s, the rapid decline in the infant mortality rate in the United States has made enormous strides largely because of NICHD-sponsored research. At the time of this writing, in the United States, the infant mortality rate now sits at about six deaths out of every thousand births, compared to twenty-five deaths out of every thousand born in 1963.

In contrast, according to the United Nations, the worldwide infant mortality rate currently averages about 50 neonatal deaths per every thousand live births. Little information is available in many countries regarding RDS specific mortality rates, though the lung disease is considered a major contributor to neonatal mortality worldwide.

Patrick's death set the groundwork for advances in neonatal respiratory care by attracting worldwide media attention at the very time when newborn care in the United States desperately needed a boost. And so it was that Patrick's death would inspire researchers and medical men who sought to minimize infant and parental suffering.

14

May Children Have Light

We can say with some assurance that, although children may be
the victims of fate, they will not be the victims of our neglect.
—John F. Kennedy, remark on signing the Maternal and Maternal
and Child Health and Mental Retardation Planning Amendments,
October 24, 1963, less than one month before his death

For the president and Mrs. Kennedy, Patrick's death produced a profound sense of loss. Emerging from the crisis of losing a baby, the president and Jackie experienced a new and intensified intimacy.

Eight weeks after Patrick's death, and five days before signing the
historic NICHD bill, President Kennedy went to Boston to attend a
Democratic fund-raising dinner. The next day, he went to a Harvard–
Columbia football game with his close friends Dave Powers and Kenneth O'Donnell.

"Toward the end of the first half," O'Donnell later recalled, "Dave
and I noticed he was unusually silent, as if his mind was far away from
the game. He turned to me and said, 'I want to go to Patrick's grave, and
I want to go there alone, with nobody from the newspapers following
me.'"[81]

---

81. O'Donnel and Powers, *"Johnny, We Hardly Knew Ye,"* 430–31.

We made our way out of the stadium to his car, with Pierre Salinger and his entourage of reporters hurrying to their cars behind us. I said a few words to a Secret Service agent, who spoke to the Boston Irish police officer in charge of the parking lot. The policeman saw to it that Salinger and the reporters did not move until the president's car was safely out of sight.

At the cemetery in Brookline, the president looked at the simple headstone with only one word, "Kennedy," inscribed upon it, and said to me, "He seems so alone here."

The president's comment would prove prophetic.

Fifteen weeks after Patrick's death, less than the time required for Mrs. Kennedy's caesarian section wound to heal, the president and first lady left the White House and journeyed to Fort Worth, Texas. The next day, the parents went on to Dallas, where America's destiny would be altered by an assassin's bullet.

Had the Kennedys been ordinary parents, it would have been justifiable for them to stay home that November day and yield to their grief. But the president and first lady belonged to the world.

Lining the roadway that historic day were thousands of passionately optimistic people, many of them young mothers and fathers holding babies and children aloft, waving at the presidential couple as they drove by, beaming with pride and hope for the future.

Most of the infants and children present that day would become parents, and it would be their newborns and generations thereafter who would reap the benefits of Patrick's short life.

Patrick's death brings to mind the words of Jesus in the Gospel of John: "In most solemn truth I tell you that unless the grain of wheat falls into the ground and dies it remains what it was—a single grain, but that if it dies it yields a rich harvest."[82]

In the end, the president would, in perhaps a loving fate, fulfill his desire that Patrick not be alone.

---

82. John 12:24, Weymouth New Testament.

The body of Patrick and that of his stillborn sister Arabella were reinterred on December 4, 1963, alongside their father at Arlington National Cemetery. There they lie, atop a grassy and gently sloping hill, near a majestic sliver of dancing light known as the eternal flame.

Behind-the-Scenes Interviews: The Three Days That Changed Everything

Interviews:

James Drorbaugh, MD, James Hughes, MD, and William Bernhard, MD

James Drorbaugh, MD
Interviewee

Michael Ryan, RRT - NPS
Interviewer

> *Dr. Drorbaugh was a forty-one-year-old instructor in the Department of Pediatrics at Harvard Medical School when he received a call requesting a clinical consult on the newly born Kennedy baby. Living with his wife of sixty-five years, Dr. Drorbaugh enjoys lunching at the local yacht club and arranging activities for those living in his retirement community.*

Nonverbatim Interview
Kaneohe, Hawaii
November 4, 2012

MR: Hello, Dr. Drorbaugh. Before we discuss the life of Patrick Bouvier Kennedy, could you tell me a little bit about your background and your formative years in clinical pediatrics?

JD: Well, I was already in premed at Princeton when the war started in 1941. While there I joined the navy V-12 program. Following graduation, I was sent by the navy to medical school, where I would graduate from the Columbia University College of Physicians and Surgeons. Bill Silverman was then the chief resident. When the war ended in 1945, we were discharged with the understanding that we would serve for two years on active duty after completing one year of an internship.

MR: What drew you to specialize in pediatrics?

JD: In 1948, while serving in the navy, I was stationed in the dispensary at the Quantico Marine Corp Base. The mothers brought their children to the Quantico dispensary for illnesses and I realized that I liked taking care of children. That's when I decided to go into pediatrics as a specialty.

MR: As a practicing physician, what bought you to the Boston Lying-in Hospital [BLI]?[83]

JD: When I left Quantico, I went to a fellowship at Rochester University School of Medicine. The fellowship was for six months in the physiology department and six months in pathology. The physiology department there had a strong interest in pulmonary physiology, which they had studied during the war. They had me do research comparing the mechanics of ventilation in animals of different size. I loved working there and after the two years of residency we moved back to Rochester where I had a combined appointment in the department of pediatrics and physiology. With the help of the physiologist, we developed a method for measuring ventilation in infants using a sensitive pressure gage in a closed box. It was because of this research that I was invited to join the Neonatal Research Lab at the Boston Lying-in Hospital. My wife and I also had strong family ties to New England and so we moved back.

---

83. In 1966, the Boston Lying-in (BLI) Hospital was renamed the Boston Hospital for Women and, in 1980, was reincorporated into the newer Brigham and Women's Hospital.

MR: Where did you do your pediatric residency?

JD: I did my pediatric residency at Boston Children's Hospital in 1950 to 1952. That residency had a rotation through the nurseries at the Boston Lying-in [located across the street from Boston Children's] as part of our training. In 1954, as mentioned earlier, I returned to the Lying-in to work in Clement A. Smith's Neonatal Research Laboratory. At that time, my focus was on pulmonary physiology in the newborn, both normal and those with respiratory distress. In 1956, I left the laboratory to go into private pediatric practice with a group of pediatricians who were also attending physicians at the BLI nursery. Our pediatric group took turns making rounds at BLI and teaching medical students and residents. I continued with this group until my family and I moved away from Boston in 1972.

MR: Could you briefly describe the culture at the Boston Lying-in Hospital at the time you were there?

JD: At the Boston Lying-in Hospital, the Neonatal Research Laboratory was established under the direction of Dr. Clement A. Smith, who, in 1946, had published a small book, *Physiology of the Newborn*. This book [the first American book on neonatology] described what was known at that time about the embryology and physiology of the various organ systems in the newborn infant, including the pulmonary and circulatory systems. Studies of the newborn were started in Boston Lying-in, Babies Hospital in New York, and other nurseries in the United States and abroad. It was this research that brought us to the point of being able to measure the pH, arterial pO_2, and the pCO_2 values as we did for the Kennedy baby.[84] That research in the early

---

84. The abbreviation pH stands for the partial pressure of hydrogen, denoting hydrogen ion concentration in the blood; pCO2 is an abbreviation for the partial pressure of carbon dioxide, a waste product of the lung; and pO2 is an abbreviation for the partial pressure of oxygen in the blood.

1950s was the beginning of all the research leading to advances in care and treatment of sick newborns now provided by newborn intensive care units [NICUs].

MR: The newborn intensive care unit I practice in today in your time was likely viewed as a distant vision by the many pioneers associated with newborn studies. What period do you think marked the shift between specialized care of the infant and our current NICUs?

JD: In my view, there was a long period of gestation before NICUs were born. This started after World War II, when pediatricians were allowed access to sick premature infants in premature nurseries.

MR: Let's talk about the day Patrick Bouvier Kennedy was born. I understand you were in your office tending to pediatric patients when you received an urgent call from Boston Children's Hospital. The caller [Dr. Jim Hughes] requested a consultation for an infant born to President and Mrs. John F. Kennedy, at the Otis Air Force Base hospital located in Cape Cod. The caller discussed the infant was born premature and in respiratory distress and you must leave right away to go see the baby. What were your first thoughts?

JD: Well, following the phone call, the first thing I did was take out the shoe shining kit I had in my desk drawer and shine my shoes. I think that was a reflex action to give myself a chance to adjust to what was going on!

MR: What happened then?

JD: I grabbed my doctor's bag and went outside and hailed a cab. We then drove to the National Guard hangar at Logan Airport where upon arrival I was met by air force staff and was flown immediately to the Otis Air Force Base hospital in Cape Cod.

MR: What happened after you landed at the Otis Air Force Base?

JD: The president met me when I stepped off the plane and said we would go to see the baby.

MR: What was your first impression of the president?

JD: To be honest, I don't think I formed any first impression of the president. Our discussion focused entirely on the baby.

MR: What was your first impression of Patrick?

JD: My impression of Patrick was that he was in significant respiratory distress. After examining him, I advised that we should transfer him to Children's Hospital.

MR: Could Patrick have been managed at Otis Air Force Base hospital just as easily as at Children's Hospital?

JD: In those days, there were no practical interventions to save the preterm baby in severe respiratory distress. Typical management would include experienced nursing personnel, a humidified isolette with oxygen as needed, and IV access to treat acidosis.[85] If improvement occurred, it would generally happen in the first few days. Many babies then diagnosed with RDS did not survive.

However, the reason for transfer to Boston Children's was the research group at Boston Lying-in Hospital, under the direction of Dr. Clement A. Smith, had developed the technique of catheterizing the umbilical artery to obtain blood for pO_2 and pCO_2, pH, and other blood tests. These measurements were used to monitor the status of the baby and, along with clinical assessment, guided therapy. We transferred Patrick to Children's so that those tests would be available to follow the clinical course.

MR: I was told the Boston Lying-in Hospital contained one of the few blood gas machines in the Boston area and became popular

---

85. Also referred to as an incubator, an isolette is a closed apparatus capable of providing, for the newborn infant, controlled temperature, humidification, and oxygen concentration. Acidosis is an acidic condition of the blood created by excess CO2 (respiratory acidosis) and/or nonvolatile acids.

among other pediatricians who would send, via taxicab, iced blood samples from nurseries all over the city.[86]

JD: I've often thought the arrival of the blood gas machine helped usher in the beginning of newborn intensive care units.

MR: How did you monitor infant oxygenation before the advent of the blood gas machine?

JD: Before we had the capacity to do blood gases, the only way to judge oxygenation was by monitoring the infant's color. One technique I remember was pressing on the baby's skin and watching the blood flow back for its color and the rapidity of return. I guess if the infant began to work harder and harder at breathing, we would assume he needed more oxygen. We didn't have mechanical ventilation.[87]

MR: In 1963, did the BLI or Boston Children's Hospital contain a NICU?

JD: There were no NICUs at either facility. Sick babies were kept in segregated areas then called the special care nursery.

MR: Tell me about the transport back to Boston with Patrick [inside his isolette] in the rear of the ambulance.

JD: The transport back to Boston was very fast, and though I was enclosed in the rear of the ambulance, I recall seeing crowds of people on nearly every overpass we went under.

MR: What occurred when you pulled into the emergency department entrance at Boston Children's Hospital?

JD: In those days there wasn't an emergency entrance to the hospital, we just drove up to the front door. A sizable crowd had gathered in front waiting for us.

---

86. A blood gas machine is a small, box-size mechanical apparatus that aspirates blood from a syringe or capillary tube and measures the pH, pCO_2, and pO_2 values of the blood.
87. Mechanical ventilation describes a mechanical ventilator that automatically cycles to give breaths to assist or replace spontaneous breathing of a patient, most often through an endotracheal tube placed directly into the trachea (windpipe).

MR: Could you describe to me what occurred at the time of admission to the hospital?

JD: Following admission to the hospital, the team from the Neonatal Research Lab at Boston Lying-in [located across the street] came to Children's and put in an umbilical catheter. Blood samples were taken, and as suspected, pO_2 was down and pCO_2 was elevated. Therapy using the incubator with added oxygen was used. X-rays were taken and we used a catheter in the umbilical vein to administer fluids and to treat acidosis as needed. The infant was considered stable at this point. Also at this time, most of the senior staff at Children's Hospital were present as well as the neonatal specialists from the Boston Lying-in.

MR: What happened the rest of the afternoon and evening?

JD: I stayed in Patrick's room observing him throughout the rest of the day and was asked to stay in the hospital overnight.

MR: How did Patrick do overnight?

JD: During the night, I was called to see the baby one time because of a brief episode of apnea. I could find nothing changed and we continued observation throughout the night into morning.

MR: What happened in the morning?

JD: In the morning [Thursday] we repeated the blood studies and, as I remember, they were about the same as the admission studies. President Kennedy came by to check on the baby. We looked at him together and I told him we would continue observation. Bob Gross, chief of surgery at Children's, with senior staff came by to tell us that the hyperbaric chamber would be available if we thought we needed it. Gross's offer was based upon his cardiac surgical team's experience using the chamber to operate on children with congenital heart disease. The thinking was that if we could keep pO_2 at reasonable levels, tissue metabolism would continue without the development of metabolic acidosis, giving hope for a few more hours leading to recovery. Since it was a therapy which had never been used to treat respiratory distress at that time, it was considered a treatment of last resort.

MR: Was endotracheal intubation discussed as an option to treat Patrick's respiratory distress?[88]

JD: I don't believe intubation or the use of mechanical ventilation was discussed as an option when the hyperbaric chamber was under consideration. We did not have the means to mechanically ventilate babies at the time. Infants then were only intubated short term in the delivery room and operating room, using hand inflation devices [bagging]. Otherwise, no infants with RDS were being intubated and mechanically ventilated in Boston at that time.

MR: I understand that in the early sixties, the hazards of intubation and mechanical ventilation of the newborn were considered so significant very few doctors were willing to attempt the treatment, and then only as a last-ditch effort.

JD: Yes, most mechanical ventilators of the time were designed for adult use and not for babies. The adult ventilators would produce high and unpredictable pressures in the infant lungs and lead to pneumothoraxes in addition to other physical hazards. The therapy was considered too risky.

MR: I understand the embryonic period of assisted mechanical ventilation of the newborn, in North America, began mostly in the early 1960s. It was during that period a few groups in San Francisco, Denver, New York, Memphis, and Toronto were making attempts to treat RDS babies using intubation with mechanical ventilation, though the therapy was usually only attempted on babies that would otherwise not survive.

JD: I wonder if the first big advance in the treatment of RDS fol-

88. Endotracheal intubation is a procedure in which a breathing tube is passed directly into the trachea (windpipe) through the mouth or, more uncommonly, the nose.

lowing Patrick's death was the development of effective assisted ventilation.

MR: Following the time of Patrick's death in 1963 from RDS, the development of ventilators tailored to newborn use really began to accelerate, culminating in 1970 with the introduction of the baby bird ventilator, the first mass-produced infant ventilator.

JD: Yes, ventilation technology took a big leap.

MR: Returning to Thursday, the day after Patrick's admission to Children's, how did he appear then?

JD: On that [Thursday] afternoon, the infant's clinical condition appeared to be worsening. His breathing was more labored and the tachypnea (rapid breathing) persisted. As I recall, the blood gases were essentially unchanged. With the worsening clinical picture, it was decided to move the infant to the hyperbaric chamber area in case his clinical condition indicated that therapy should be tried.

MR: Whose decision was it to use the hyperbaric chamber?

JD: To the best of my recollection, it was a group consensus. Bob Gross suggested the chamber as a means of oxygenating Patrick if he failed to maintain his oxygenation on his own. Alex Nadas [pediatric cardiologist] was involved, in addition to a couple others whose names I cannot recall. I was in favor of trying. I don't remember hearing any objections from anyone pertaining to the chamber's use. We simply had nothing else to offer to Patrick in the way of therapy. We finally moved Patrick to the room containing the chamber in case it would be needed. After the move to the hyperbaric chamber area, his clinical condition worsened and it was decided to try the chamber.

MR: In the fact intubation and mechanical ventilation to treat RDS was apparently then such an unproven therapy, it's clear to me how the decision was made to go with the chamber. I was told intubation of the RDS infant at that time was performed on infants who otherwise would die and there were simply no other life-saving interventions. How did Patrick look following the move to the area containing the hyperbaric chamber?

JD: Continued observation after the move to the hyperbaric area indicated that his clinical condition was getting worse. Breathing was more labored with severe retractions. His skin color was not as good. At that point, it was decided to try the hyperbaric chamber to attempt to stabilize his condition so recovery could proceed. As I remember it, Dr. Bernhard [pediatric cardiothoracic surgeon], a technician whose name I cannot recall, Dr. Bob Smith [pediatric anesthesiologist], and I went into the chamber with Patrick. Outside the chamber were other technicians and a small group [about four or five] of senior physicians on the staff of Children's. President Kennedy soon arrived, and Dr. Levine joined them after he arrived from New York. We could communicate with them by phone and they could see us through the port. The chamber was pressurized and we continued to observe Patrick. Initially there were some indications he was improving, but that did not last long. Thereafter, it became progressively hard to keep Patrick oxygenated. Within a few hours, he had another more prolonged period of apnea, at which point he was intubated by Dr. Smith, who then proceeded to hand bag [ventilate] the baby for a number of hours. Following placement of the breathing tube, Patrick's work of breathing became somewhat decreased, although he continued to clinically deteriorate. Continued observation during the night showed no improvement with a downhill course, which ended in death early [4:04 A.M.] Friday morning. We told his father.

MR: What occurred immediately after Patrick's death?

JD: After Patrick died, he remained inside while we waited several hours to decompress the chamber before we could come out. The Children's Hospital staff who had been with us when we went into the chamber stayed to support us as we waited for the chamber to be decompressed and met us when we came out. They thanked us for our efforts and wanted us to know they shared our sorrow at not being able to save Patrick. The president was not there when we came out. I don't know what he did after Patrick died. We shared our feelings of sadness with the senior staff, and then we went our separate ways. Our home is within walking distance of Children's Hospital, so I walked home. It was daylight by then.

MR: What occurred after your arrival home?

JD: Later that morning the president phoned me to thank me for trying to help his son. I told him how sorry we were that we had not been able to save Patrick. His reply was, "It wasn't in the cards." After fifty years of thinking about it, this seems to me to be the best summary of what happened.

MR: Besides your initial conversation with Mrs. Kennedy at the Otis hospital, did you speak to her following Patrick's death?

JD: No, I did not, although a week or two later, I got a small framed portrait [picture included in book] of the White House signed by the first lady and, again, thanking us for our efforts. I believe others of us who participated received this portrait as well.

MR: Only days following the death of Patrick, you received a letter from Pierre Salinger [President Kennedy's press secretary] requesting input upon setting up a special fund for RDS research. The letter appears to be the first documented exchange between the medical establishment and a presidential administration official regarding funding for RDS research. What were your thoughts when you responded to Salinger's request?

JD: Salinger's letter was received at a time many of us in the newborn medical community felt frustration at not being able to do more for Patrick or any of the newborns with RDS. So when he personally asked me about setting up a government-sponsored fund, it sure seemed like a great opportunity to get significant funding for neonatal research benefiting every aspect of newborn care, especially RDS.

MR: What stands as the most memorable part of the entire Kennedy baby ordeal?

JD: The part of the story that means the most to me is the role played by the president and the first lady, the grace with which they handled an unexpected crisis, which ended with the death of their newborn son. It was a very tragic episode made more bearable because of their graciousness towards all of us every step of the way. This is the main thing I would like those who read your story to remember.

MR: Thank you, Dr. Drorbaugh.

William F. Bernhard, MD, FACS
Interviewee

Michael Ryan, RRT - NPS
Interviewer

> *Dr. Bill Bernhard, a member of Dr. Bob Gross's pioneering pediatric open-heart team, arranged for the experimental (and then practical) use of the hyperbaric chamber to perform pediatric open-heart surgery. The chamber, known to force large amounts of oxygen into the body, was ultimately used to treat Patrick Bouvier Kennedy. Dr. Bernhard discusses his involvement with the hyperbaric and its use in Patrick's treatment. Living in the Boston area with his wife, Bernhard enjoys working around the house and, when able, going out in his sailboat.*

Nonverbatim Interview
Boston, Massachusetts
March 19, 2013

MR: Hello, Dr. Bernhard. You are an important figure in the use of utilizing cardiac surgical techniques inside the hyperbaric chamber. Could you describe to me the use of the hyperbaric chamber in the repair of congenital heart defects in 1963? I would also like to discuss its association in the treatment of Patrick Bouvier Kennedy.

WB: Let's first begin the discussion by putting the hyperbaric chamber and its use within the context of my clinical research program in pediatric cardiac surgery. The project had nothing to do with infant lung disease, and in fact, we tried to avoid any patients with problems of the lungs because of the possibility of lung injury. I was always afraid of a tension pneumothorax caused by ruptured blebs.[89] Many cardiac babies back then that were born and re-suscitated very vigorously could rupture during decompression. We mostly never saw blebs unless there was resuscitative damage ahead of time.

Because I was definitely afraid of lung injury, babies placed inside the tank would receive a chest X-ray to rule out lung disease and bleb formation. Even staff members who worked inside the tank had a chest X-ray to rule out silent lung disease. So we were absolutely not involved with any pulmonary problems at all.

MR: Can you discuss some background about the hyperbaric chamber?

WB: Well, the hyperbaric facility was located within the industrial medicine division of the building housing the Harvard School of Public Health. At four hundred dollars a month, I was able to lease it for a number of months. If they were not using it for teaching or any other reasons, I was able to conduct animal and clinical experiments inside the tank. So certain cardiac surgical procedures were being carried out inside the hyperbaric tank in addition to being used to conduct other experiments involving O_2 [oxygen] and CO_2 [carbon dioxide] measurements under pressure at two to three atmospheres absolute.

Again, we were staying away from pulmonary disease be-cause of the difficulty in preventing complications like inter-stitial pulmonary hemorrhage, alveolar capillary block, and so on; we saw some instances in puppies that we placed inside the tank on 100 percent oxygen with three atmospheres absolute of pressure. So that's the background.

MR: What was the benefit of performing operations inside the tank?

WB: Up until this time [before the use of the hyperbaric chamber], we were unable to force additional oxygen into plasma solu-

89. Blebs (or bullae) are small air pockets that form inside or on (subpleural) the surface of the lung, often created by ruptured alveoli.

tion on 100 percent oxygen, and this was the key objective. The hyperbaric chamber helped us to do a little of that. Unless you have alveolar–capillary function, significant oxygen transfer cannot occur. So we were happily doing our clinical research program operating on babies inside the tank and began accomplishing some of the goals I was interested in.

MR: So you were aware that any disruption of gas exchange at the alveolar capillary level would eliminate getting oxygen to the red cell mass.

WB: Yes, and there were other things to consider as well. An obstruction of a small bronchus could result in a bleb that if ruptured during chamber decompression would cause a tension pneumothorax. My experience with these newborn babies is that by the time you inserted chest tubes and evacuated the air, and hooked them up to the bottles to reexpand their lungs, you might have a dead baby. I was very careful about tackling pulmonary problems.

MR: So once inside the pressurized chamber, it was not uncommon to encounter infants with underlying pulmonary blebs placing them at risk for tension pneumothorax?

WB: Well, we are mainly speaking of babies placed in the chamber following vigorous resuscitation. As you know, excessive positive pressure transmitted via the endotracheal tube to the airway could create subpleural blebs in the lungs, causing those lungs to collapse [pneumothorax]. Some infants with cardiac problems I received were resuscitated in this fashion. Some had [alveolar] ruptures, which would result in collapsed lung segments as seen on X-ray. As I said, though, I was not dealing with babies who had primary pulmonary problems. I was dealing with babies who had congenital heart disease.

MR: I know that you had performed cardiac surgery on approximately a hundred babies inside the hyperbaric chamber. More importantly, your work resulted in nice outcomes for most of those infants.

WB: Well, we were looking for methods to improve the cardiac surgical outcomes for babies in our hospital. We believed many of the cardiac babies would benefit with an open operative intervention if we had a few extra minutes during inflow occlusions,[90] and so we were looking for ways to accomplish this objective. Physiologically, we were seeking to temporarily increase the arterial pO_2, [in acyanotic patients] up to a thousand to provide a few extra minutes of inflow occlusion time.[91] These high pO_2s could not be held for very long, and you could burn up the oxygen fast with the circulation interrupted. The tank provided the mode that made possible these high pO_2s, at least for a few minutes of time.

Now a few minutes may not seem like much, but you can do lot of work in that time. Again, optimizing oxygen content in the plasma was the objective. It was a way of providing a little extra time for the operation. My interest was buying a few extra minutes to perform the surgery. Furthermore, you could gain more time by decreasing the baby's core temperature, so hypothermia was very important. For this reason we dropped the temperature in these babies to about thirty-three to thirty-five degrees centigrade in order to protect the brain and central nervous system.

MR: What were some of the more common cardiac operations you performed inside the tank?

WB: Well, besides creating ASDs [atrial septal defects] in transposition [of the great vessels] cases, we were also doing a number of valve openings in aortic and pulmonary stenosis. We devised simple techniques that were effective in these cases. You could accomplish these procedures quickly and restore the circulation. We did many cases without any evidence of central nervous system difficulty. Most of these cases would pan out as long as you

---

90. Inflow occlusion is the temporary occlusion of the inferior and superior vena cava.
91. Known as the PaO2, this symbol refers to the partial pressure of oxygen in arterial blood.

had good pulmonary blood flow, with normal alveolar–capillary membrane gas [O_2 and CO_2] transfer.

MR: As a side note, infant cooling has recently enjoyed resurgence as a postresuscitative treatment for newborn infant asphyxia, helping to retard potential damage to the brain.

WB: We knew then cooling the baby under certain operative conditions would support the central nervous system by reducing oxygen utilization by the brain.

MR: In the early 1960s, little was available to support the [noncardiac] preterm baby in respiratory distress. I understand there were a few physicians around at the time that would attempt to intubate and ventilate the preterm baby, choosing to try it on those who would have died otherwise from respiratory distress syndrome. I also understand at that time, if the baby did not die from RDS, he would probably succumb from the complications [primarily pneumothoraxes] created by excessive pressure pumped into the lungs following intubation and mechanical ventilation.[92]

WB: Oh absolutely. We were very aware of this and also the amount of dead space in the adult ventilator circuit, an amount exceeding the capacity of the infant lungs. In my work, we never used any ventilators on babies inside the operating room. We used an anesthesia bag connected to an endotracheal tube and the right hand of an anesthetist that was very skilled in manual ventilation.

MR: Tell me about the day when Patrick Bouvier Kennedy arrived at the hospital.

WB: Well, I was in my laboratory minding my own business when I got a call from [Jim] Drorbaugh. He mentioned he had a baby in severe respiratory distress that was a member of an important

---

92. During Patrick Bouvier Kennedy's time, the risks of mechanical ventilation were commonly viewed as being so dangerous that doctors would avoid its use unless the infant could not otherwise survive.

family known to the overseers of the hospital. He then asked me if I could do something with him to help the baby, asking me to come over and take a look at him.

I can remember saying, "Hey, this infant's in respiratory distress and I don't want any part of it." [laughs] And he said, "Ahhh, come over and have a look anyway." Well, I walked over there to this Harvard Industrial Medicine facility [Harvard School of Public Health] which projected out into the Prouty Garden of the hospital. By the time I got over there, there were many physicians gathered around, the chief of pediatric medicine and a number of other hospital staff. It became obvious they were having difficulty stabilizing this premature infant. By this time the baby had been in the hospital a number of hours. He was in significant respiratory distress and they felt they were losing and were willing to try another course of treatment. And this is about where I fit in. So at this point, I couldn't possibly refuse not to get involved, and that was it.

MR: So Jim basically gave you a call telling you he had a premature infant in significant RDS and needed help.

WB: Yeah, that's right. He mentioned he had a newborn patient he picked up at a hospital in Cape Cod and brought back to Boston; so they were trying to help him. When I arrived on the scene, everybody present was unable to provide help. He was a premature baby who looked in rough shape, working really hard to breathe.

MR: So by the time you saw this infant, he was working really hard to breathe and appeared in full-blown respiratory failure?

WB: Absolutely! Nobody in attendance was able to initiate any clinical progress, so we took him inside the tank and pressurized. Within a few moments, we saw an improvement in the EKG pattern, probably an ST segment elevation, but it was obvious to me after a very few minutes we were not going to be able to help the baby, and that's what I told the baby's father: "I think we're not going to be able to provide help for the little boy." I also said that if we had to insert a breathing tube into the infant's trachea [intubate] and ventilate with 100 percent oxygen that would indicate further deterioration. Any time you were forced to intubate these little babies at this stage they were on their way out. It was a desperate and difficult situation, and placement in the pressurized tank was a desperate measure.

MR: That's what Jim [Drorbaugh] told me. He said there were simply no effective means to treat premature babies in severe RDS, and the use of the tank, in this case, was simply a last-ditch trial of therapy.

WB: We had no previous clinical experience either. Putting RDS babies inside the hyperbaric chamber under normal circumstances is something I would have not done. But because of the situation and the high-profile nature of the case, with the parents, and the political situation, that's how I got involved. We definitely avoided pulmonary disease in infants.

MR: Did you talk often to the baby's father?

WB: Oh, sure, several times.

MR: And what did he have to say?

WB: Well, I won't go into that with detail but he understood with one look at the baby what the problem was, and after a few hours he knew we were not accomplishing anything. And I told him we were not accomplishing anything. He was very concerned and pleasant in nature. We had a number of chats.

MR: Now I know Jim [Drorbaugh] was the primary attending physician. Was he also the primary liaison between the baby and the president?

WB: Oh, yeah, Jim picked the baby up from a local hospital [Otis Air Force Base hospital] and had been conversing with the baby's father and other staff.

MR: Did the baby's father enter the tank at any time?

WB: No, he did not go inside the tank. There was Drorbaugh, the anesthetist, a technician, the baby, and myself, and that was it. It [the tank] was not open to participation by lot of people. It was a very cramped space.

MR: Who was the anesthetist?

WB: I don't remember, though he was very good. He slipped the tube [intubate] in the baby inside the tank and began ventilating [bagging] the baby. That's when things were slipping away.

MR: Jim Drorbaugh also stated to me the baby began to exhibit apneic spells inside the tank. The baby's impending respiratory failure as you describe at that moment appears to coincide with his apneic spells requiring the need for intubation.

WB: Absolutely. It was obvious he was not going to last long unless we put a tube in and we kept trying. At that time, intubation was a last resort, and you could almost be assured you were going to lose a baby when it got to that point.

MR: Why did they not intubate the baby initially before trying the tank?

WB: Well, initially the baby appeared to be holding his own inside the isolette containing 100 percent oxygen. The treatment protocol for premature babies with RDS was then well established. That would be a well-moisturized isolette containing a set percentage of oxygen. You just had to be there constantly monitoring for signs of deterioration. Back then, you would almost never start out intubating a baby unless death was imminent and no other choice was available. Unless they were doing badly and really struggling, you would not do that.

MR: Now because of the family situation and the fact the president was standing nearby, did this produce extra pressure on the staff?

WB: Well, some political tension was there, but it did not change our actions. We would not have done anything differently. The only difference was that I was there as a favor to Dr. Drorbaugh. Otherwise, this was a routine pressurization treatment inside the hyperbaric. Everything was quiet and businesslike.

MR: What was the expression on the president's face? Did you notice sadness, despair, concern, or tears?

WB: Well, just like all parents, he was very concerned. That's what you would expect. He was a good parent and a wonderful father, and you could tell that. He was very concerned. And this is something you would expect. He was very cooperative and knowledgeable, and picked up things very fast. He was a quick study.

MR: Whose idea was it to put the baby in the chamber?

WB: Well, it certainly wasn't mine! It was probably a collective decision by senior staff. Drorbaugh and I had done some experiments together and he knew we were careful about excluding anyone that did not have a normal chest X-ray. We had never placed an infant inside the chamber for any pulmonary problems. This was a first. My point is that I was cooperating with everyone else because everyone was trying so hard to save this baby. I would say the decision was made to put the baby inside the chamber because they were losing and wanted to try everything possible, even though we had no experience treating RDS in the tank.

MR: Well, we know what happened to the baby, his father, and everyone else. How were you affected by the loss of the baby? Tell me a little bit about how you felt after Patrick died.

WB: Well, in cardiac surgery we would occasionally lose patients. Inwardly, we knew we had done our best, and when everything proceeds according to plan, you still lose a few patients. This is especially true when everyone puts forth a maximum effort and we made a maximum effort with this baby [Patrick]. We just employed a technique never before used, only because there was nothing left to do. So when a child dies following every attempt to save him, life must go on.

MR: In my twenty-three years of clinical experience within a high-acuity, level 3, inner-city [Los Angeles] neonatal intensive care unit, throughout that period, I have been exposed to quite a few newborn deaths. As both clinician and being human, I do recognize I am forced into accepting the fact that despite the best treatment possible, infants will sometimes die. We often refer to such infants as God's babies.

This leads me to ask the following question. Given the political tension involved with the patient being the son of a popular U.S. president, did you feel any personal guilt or shame or a feeling that if you would have to do it over, would have done things differently?

WB: Well, no, because I knew the situation was desperate. I told him [the president] the baby was probably going to die. I had to later tell him [the president] we were going to have to put an endotracheal tube in, and those were my final words to him [the president]. I basically never saw him again after that. I never talked to him again or had any contact with the White House at all about any part of this.

MR: Well, basically when you first saw the baby [Patrick] and you went into the tank, you took one look at him and pretty much knew the baby was desperately ill.

WB: Absolutely. This was a desperate move. The other medical group [Clement Smiths] supposedly knew a lot about prematurity and RDS. As I mentioned, the Harvard School of Public Health owned the tank and permitted numerous animal and clinical studies to be carried out. As mentioned, I was renting the tank for my own studies from the Harvard School of Industrial Medicine. Other studies in industrial medicine were also being undertaken at the time, so there were a lot of reasons to go the last mile. And if the same situation had came up with another baby, we would make it very clear to a parent that we in general were avoiding any patients with pulmonary disease. This was not new information.

MR: Do you know what was said to the president before going into the tank?

WB: No, I do not know what occurred before I got there. When I got there, we didn't delay therapy and within a few minutes went inside the hyperbaric chamber and pressurized at three point zero ATA. It appeared for a few minutes we were making some progress, but after that it was downhill. As I said, it was all about getting oxygen into the blood and that was the key. With infant RDS, that would be a hard thing to do [take oxygen into the blood]. The hyperbaric might buy a few minutes of time as long as you had some alveolar–capillary function.

MR: When the baby died, who told the president?

WB: I don't remember, it's been so long ago.

MR: Can you tell me anything about other members of the pediatric and neonatal staff?

WB: There was probably a lot of tension and weight on the other side [pediatric staff] in terms of doing the proper thing. A Kennedy family pediatrician [Dr. Levine] contacted by the family showed up putting pressure on the other pediatricians, increasing their stress level. He showed up at a time when the baby, and I'm not sure why, began to show some signs of fleeting hope, but it didn't last very long.

MR: Regardless of anyone else, how were you affected by the baby's death?

WB: Never talked to anyone else about it after that, especially the media. We did not provide any information to anyone. Whether the hospital did or did not [provide information about the baby], I didn't pay any attention to it. But I don't think the hospital knew anything because others involved in the baby's care did not talk to any hospital spokesmen or anybody else. I certainly didn't give any, in the media or at any time for fifty years. This is my first mention of it. Nobody said anything about it. It was an experimental procedure, and that was the end of it.

MR: Following the death of Patrick Bouvier Kennedy, the event bought hyaline membrane disease into the public spotlight. What appeared to be a direct consequence of his death was a tremendous spike in newborn lung research. Fifty years later, many people still refer to RDS as the disease that killed the Kennedy baby.

WB: That's good, because it was an area that needed a lot of clinical research attention. I was very involved in many other things at that time, and infant lung disease was not one of them, so I never paid attention to lung research after that. As I said, I just got roped in to help out, because I was asked to help out.

MR: You were a pediatric heart surgeon during a period when the mortality rate among infants and children was much higher as compared to now. How was it telling parents their child was nearing death, or died?

WB: Well, among most parents there was a certain resignation to having a very sick infant, they seemed to be able to take one look and get the big picture. A lot of parents suffered silently. Most of these things I never saw too much because we never lost many babies we operated on.

MR: Did you vote for President Kennedy?

WB: Probably not. [laughs] I voted Republican. But we had some things in common; we were both naval officers in the war and happened to be in some of the same areas at different times. Both of us were dads, too.

MR: What do you remember most about the president on that day?

WB: I remember him most as a very congenial, pleasant father and a very quick study as to what was going on. He picked up things fast. We had many brief conversations about the baby and he stayed out of the way. He had a lot of people around him. I remember his brother Teddy being around, and Pierre Salinger, the press secretary, seemed to be a constant presence. Everybody stayed in the background, so there was no problem. The whole scene was pretty low key, although it was a very tough situation.

MR: You were inside the tank when the baby died.

WB: Yes, absolutely. I never left and could not even possibly leave that situation because nobody knew enough [about the hyperbaric chamber] about what needed to be done. So I stayed there. We had a monitor on the baby and so when everything came to a halt, the anesthetist stopped bagging and took the tube out and that was that.

MR: So when the baby died, did you stay in the tank to decompress follow his death?

WB: We did have to decompress to let people in to take care of things. It was no big deal, and I just left at that point.

MR: When the baby died, was the father told at that moment over the intercom or did you go outside the tank to tell him?

BB: At that point I don't remember what was said. I do remember telling the father a half-hour earlier we were losing and so he knew we were losing and so he was prepared. It was important there were no shocks to anybody.

MR: Do you ever miss performing cardiac surgery, the intellectual engagement, the excitement of research, and its challenges?

WB: Well, I served in World War II in addition to my years operating so I've had enough excitement. I'm pushing ninety [years old] so the motto is staying alive; this makes life much less confusing. [laughs] I get excited going out in my sailboat, so as long as I'm able, and breathing, that's what I'm going to do.

MR: Thank you, Dr. Bernhard.

James Hughes, MD
Interviewee

Michael Ryan, RRT - NPS
Interviewer

> *In summer 1963, James Hughes, MD, was a co-pediatric resident at Boston Children's Hospital when he admitted Patrick Bouvier Kennedy for further care, and he would later sign Patrick's death certificate. A 1960 Harvard Medical School graduate, Dr. Hughes's distinguished career in medicine and public health spans a lifetime. He currently maintains a wide range of interests that include singing bass in popular operatic ensembles.*

Nonverbatim Interview
West Fairlee, Vermont
November 13, 2012

MR: Dr. Hughes, could you tell me a little about your position and what happened at the Boston Children's Hospital on the afternoon of August 7, 1963?

JH: I was in my fourth year of residency and serving as chief resident. The chief resident job was split between my colleague John Green and me. As chief residents, the two of us would alternate between the pediatric outpatient department and inpatient services. On that day, John Green was in charge of outpatient services and I was covering inpatient services and new admissions.

MR: What happened when you received the call from the Otis hospital regarding the Kennedy baby?

JH: Well, it was an ordinary busy day. The call came in as simply one of many that I would routinely receive throughout the day. I simply answered the page and the gentleman caller identified himself as Mrs. Kennedy's obstetrician [Dr. John Walsh] based in Washington, D.C. The caller explained that both he and she [Mrs. Kennedy] were currently up in Cape Cod where Mrs. Kennedy went into labor while vacationing. The caller proceeded to explain that Mrs. Kennedy's baby was born prematurely with breathing difficulties, and he requested an immediate pediatric consult and transfer to Children's. The caller was brief and he stuck with the facts. Following a short conversation in order to work out some details, the phone call then ended.

MR: What were your first thoughts following the phone call?

JH: I must admit my first thought was that perhaps it was a hoax. I quickly called my wife at home to ask her if Jackie was pregnant and she said yes. I then notified the admissions office and the chief of services to let them know we would be receiving a very special patient. I then called Jim Drorbaugh.

MR: How did you know Jim Drorbaugh?

JH: I knew Jim as an attending pediatric physician. As both an academic and practicing pediatrician in private practice, Jim was highly respected among residents at both Boston Children's and Boston City Hospital.

MR: So Jim was on call?

JH: I don't believe so. When a call comes in from the outside without an attending physician, it would become my choice whom to call. Under these unique circumstances, it became my choice to call Jim Drorbaugh. My decision was based upon his clinical newborn expertise and impeccable esteem among residents inside Boston Children's and the Boston City Hospital. I felt Jim would be the best choice to attend the president's baby.

MR: When you called Dr. Drorbaugh, do you remember his reaction?

JH: I remember it very clearly. Dr. Drorbaugh received my phone call while in his nearby office. I explained the situation to him, presenting the facts in a minimal amount of words, describing how the baby appeared [as described to me by Walsh] to be in significant respiratory distress. I then asked if he would be willing to be the physician of record and prepare for departure to see the baby and accompany the infant's return to Children's.

MR: What happened then?

JH: Well, understand that Jim was a real gentleman and just a wonderful person, and he responded to my request with a stammer in his voice [mimicking stammer] [laughs]. His first words were, "Well, I've got a lot of patients in the office and I'm not sure if I can leave right away." [laughs] This led me to believe my request did not immediately sink in. The gravity of the call must have soon been realized because he finally found a way for those patients to be taken care of so he could attend to the newborn son of the president of the United States. [laughs]

MR: What happened then following the conversation with Dr. Drorbaugh?

JH: I again called the chief of hospital services. Following that call, I then contacted all the pertinent departments in the hospital to forewarn them of the Kennedy baby's arrival. I wanted to make sure I was covered from the top on down. At the time, Dr. Louis Diamond, second in command and vice chair of the hospital staff, was filling in for the chief of the hospital, who was away on a trip.[93] Though known as an excellent pediatric generalist, Louie's—and I would never call him such to his face—specialty was hematology.

MR: Following the baby's arrival, were there any amusing anecdotes you remember against the gravity of this monumental crisis?

JH: The one and only piece of humor after the baby arrived occurred when Dr. Levine, an old Kennedy family doctor and trusted pediatrician, entered the hospital basement [Levine was picked

---

93. Dr. Diamond is often called the "Founding Father of Pediatric Hematology."

up by a police car in his New York neighborhood and hurriedly flown to Boston] stepping into an observation area outside the hyperbaric chamber. Things with the baby were looking particularly good at that point. Standing in the observation area beside the chamber at the time were the president and hospital senior staff, all of whom greeted the elderly physician. Dr. Levine then began to recount his journey from the New York area to the basement of the hospital, commenting how incredibly fast he had been brought to the location. He then began looking at his wristwatch and mentioned, "I'm very impressed with the efficiency of government!" The president with a smile and without hesitation responded, "It's about time you doctors learned that!" clearly referring to the well-publicized debate regarding the AMA's [American Medical Association's] resistance to any government intervention, a debate that continues today!

MR: What were your impressions of the president's reaction to Patrick's course at the time?

JH: The president showed concern and self-control and remained pretty cool and calm throughout, asking appropriate questions as any concerned parent would.

MR: Did you talk to the president?

JH: I talked to him very briefly before the baby arrived to Boston Children's. I was carrying the pager and received a call when someone came on the line who asked, "Dr. Hughes, are you the chief resident responsible for the Kennedy baby's admission?" I said, "Yes, I am." The caller then said, "The president of the United States wishes to speak with you," and suddenly the president was on the line. He asked me what the status was, and I said to him, "The baby is in transit and we are in the process of preparing a room for admission." I further explained that we knew he was in respiratory distress, we knew his weight, and that he was stable at that point.

MR: Were you nervous when speaking with him?

JH: I was more respectful and aware of the pressure upon him as a father having a sick baby.

MR: What was your style in managing a baby with hyaline membrane disease, or as we call it nowadays respiratory distress syndrome?

JH: My first year after graduation from Harvard Medical School [1960] had been spent as an intern in internal medicine at Massachusetts General Hospital, with minimal experience with newborns. The vagaries of subsequent pediatric schedules at Boston City and Children's had by chance been somewhat light on what today we would call the subspecialty of neonatology. It would be presumptive of me to say I had a mature "management style" but my philosophy of care was in no way unique: absolute minimal intervention. There simply were not a lot of cards to play then with a preterm HMD baby. This brings me to recall that during my first-year residency [then called internship] at Mass General, I developed an interest in pediatrics. A Harvard pediatrics star, Sidney Gellis of Boston City Hospital, became my mentor and encouraged me to do my second postgraduation year at City. He told me there I would be exposed to a more compromised and at-risk population, one that was far more subject to the acute illnesses that in large part stem from poverty and neglect. He further explained the experience would be vital before going to a major referral center such as Children's Hospital. I followed that advice and did my junior assistant resident pediatric rotation at Boston City.

There I discovered at Boston City that the basic management of a preemie, although I hesitate to use this term, was "benign neglect," which is pretty much what it was. There I discovered there was little more you could do other than keep the preemie in a nice, warm, near-sterile environment and employ feedings, along with adequate hydration and adequate amounts of oxygen inside the isolette. We did have a special incubator room where preemies were kept. This was staffed with nurses skilled in preemie handling techniques. Otherwise, there was precious little in the way of other interventions.

So I had had no real training in what would now be called the NICU simply because we did not have a NICU at Boston City Hospital. I then moved to Boston Children's where we did not have a formal NICU either. There we had a specially designated area housing sick babies, being mostly surgical patients and those transferred from area hospitals.

The big obstetric hospital in the area was the Boston Lying-in Hospital (BLIH), now called the Brigham and Women's Hospital on the Harvard campus just two blocks away. This is where most of your academic thinking was going on in preterm care and lung disease, under the direction of Clement Smith [professor of pediatrics at the BLIH Hospital, Harvard Medical School]. The BLIH facility as well did not have a NICU. However, what the BLIH facility did contain was a fairly new blood gas machine capable of determining values based on relatively small sample amounts.[94]

It was little realized then that ten years later there would be monumental technical leaps in newborn care, in addition to NICUs nationwide.

MR: What can you remember about the events which occurred leading up to the decision to place Patrick in the hyperbaric chamber?

JH: I recall the curve of Patrick's arterial blood gases appeared to be

---

94. The (small-volume) blood gas machine at BLI was reputedly the only one in town. Former personnel recall taxicabs dropping off infant blood gas samples from facilities citywide for blood gas value determination. This was a new technology, though Dr. Hughes mentions that he had performed blood gas determinations on large physiology lab samples while in medical school; it was not until the Kennedy baby came along that he first witnessed an infant blood gas determination. When he moved to Hitchcock (now Dartmouth Hitchcock Medical Center) in 1967, there were no blood gas machines suitable for repeated neonatal sampling.

deteriorating when the decision was made by the neonatology team to place Patrick in the chamber.

And mind you, we were getting flooded with calls from all around the world offering clinical advice. They would say, "Did you try this?" and "You should try that" or "You ought to do this," and so on. A tremendous influx of unsolicited input from everyone imaginable.

MR: How did other people worldwide find out so fast? What sort of media coverage did you notice while inside the hospital?

JH: Well, the media coverage was just tremendous. I do not know for sure, but I'm certain the coverage began there at the Otis hospital with press helicopters probably following the ambulance to the hospital. From there it just intensified. The executive director of the hospital at the time, Leonard Cronkhite, directed me not to speak to the press, a direction which I certainly respected. During the whole time, I believe I was quoted just once when pressured by one of the news magazines for a comment and I responded in a very dismissive way, "Ask the front office," or with words to that effect!

MR: What more could you tell me about the presence of the newspaper and television media?

JH: Well, the media pressure continued to intensify, though members of the press were strictly kept off limits from the hospital. The first night, a photographer standing atop one of the buildings down the street, using a telescopic lens, snapped a photo of me through the window while I was standing there observing the Kennedy baby. That picture wound up on the cover of *Life* magazine the following week. The photo seemed to capture a very stark and tension-filled moment in Patrick's course. The photo caption read something like, "the window an anxious nation watched."

MR: I have sitting on my bookshelf the August 16, 1963, issue of

Life magazine where you are seen standing looking over the baby as photographed through the window. I also noted there is no article attached to the photo series inside, and now I realize why! No one told them [the press] anything! Incidentally, I was struck how everyone gowned and masked when entering Patrick's room.

JH: Gown and masking, not necessarily gloving, was standard infection precautions at the time when entering a premature nursery and even the well baby nursery.

MR: Did Patrick receive antibiotics [routine for today's NICU admissions] upon admission, for presumed sepsis?

JH: No, actually there had been a recent and very sad experience in starting babies routinely on antibiotics. You may already know this, the chloramphenicol story.[95] Physicians were burnt on that so much it was quite obvious what we had done creating what was called the "gray baby syndrome" and it was still very large in everyone's mind. Routine administration of antibiotics then stopped.

Under the right circumstances, chloramphenicol was a darn good drug. I mourned its passing. At the time, there were not a lot of antibiotic options. You were left with penicillin. We did not have amoxicillin or ampicillin. We had streptomycin, but we got some auditory nerve damage out of that one. We also had the sulfonamides that also caused problems, so there was no big enthusiasm using antibiotics unless there was a very strong suspicion of sepsis.

MR: Did Patrick receive any drugs?

JH: He probably received bicarb, though it's hard to recall.

MR: What else was done with Patrick's care?

JH: As you know, he was initially in the isolette receiving oxygen;

---

95. In the late 1950s, it was discovered that the routine administration of chloramphenicol involved severe side effects, causing injury to the baby.

we monitored him with minimal care while following the blood gases. He probably received bicarb to manage acid–base balance, though nothing more. Following signs of physical deterioration, the decision was made by senior staff to move the baby to the hyperbaric chamber. I believe this was a rational choice. There were simply not a lot of cards to play when the preterm baby began to go south.

MR: Before Patrick was moved to the chamber, how did you decide which room to put Patrick in following his admission to the hospital, and how did it appear inside?

JH: The room Patrick was placed was one we hastily arranged, I believe on the fifth or sixth floor. It was in fact a makeshift private care unit, very simple, and about the size of a large kitchen. Inside was enough space for the isolette and room for about six people with one door and one window. It was through that window the picture of myself was taken and wound up on the cover of *Life* magazine.

MR: How did you feel when the baby died?

JH: I signed the death certificate.

MR: One of my final questions, we know what happened to the baby and to the Kennedy family. What happened to you, and how were you transformed by the experience?

JH: Well, a month or two after the episode, the chief of pediatrics, who had a Hopkins [Johns Hopkins University] connection, approached me about going to India. He mentioned Hopkins had a project in [Calcutta] India. Although the project was completely unassociated with my recent experience with the Kennedy baby, they thought it would be a good fit. Well, the [Kennedy] baby was lost in August, and shortly afterwards the president was shot in November. And so a month or two after that, when I arrived in Calcutta, I soon realized the death of the president hit people over there as much as it did here. People

grieved his death worldwide. When others found out I was associated with the family and pediatricians there identified me
as having been with the baby, they attached to me an aura not
unlike one they would attach to a visiting dignitary. Thereafter,
I was accompanied by an aura associated with my connection to
the baby and family, and it was palpable.

MR: Thank you, Dr. Hughes.

Bibliography

Avery, M. E., and J. Mead. "Surface Properties in Relation to Atelectasis and Hyaline Membrane Disease." *American Journal of Diseases of Children* 97 (1959): 517–23.

Baccalari, Eduardo, and Richard A. Polin, eds. *The Newborn Lung: Neonatology Questions and Controversies.* Philadelphia: Saunders Elsevier, 2008.

Baker, Jeffrey P. *The Machine in the Nursery.* Baltimore: The Johns Hopkins University Press, 1996.

Behrman, Richard E., and Adrienne Stith Butler, eds., *Preterm Birth: Causes, Consequences, and Prevention.* Washington, DC: National Academies Press, 2007.

Bengt, Robertson, Lambert M. G. Van Golde, and Joseph J. Batenburg, eds. *Pulmonary Surfactant: From Molecular Biology to Clinical Practice.* Amsterdam: Elsevier Science, 1992.

Berton, Pierre. *The Dionne Years: A Thirties Melodrama.* New York: W. W. Norton, 1978.

Blaine, Gerald, with Lisa McCubbin. *The Kennedy Detail.* New York: Gallery Books, 2010.

Bolt, R. A. *The Mortalities of Infancy.* Philadelphia: Saunders, 1923.

Brownlow, John. *The History and Design of the Foundling Hospital with a Memoir of the Founder.* London: W. and H. S. Warr, 1858.

Burton, George G., and John E. Hodgkin. *Respiratory Care—A Guide to Clinical Practice.* Philadelphia: J. B. Lippincott, 1984.

Clements, J. A. "Surface Tension of Lung Extracts." *Proceedings of the Society for Experimental Biology and Medicine* 95 (1957): 170–72.

———. "Lung Surface Tension and Surfactant: The Early Years." In *Respiratory Physiology, People and Ideas,* edited by John B. West. New York: Published for the American Physiological Society by Oxford University Press, 1996.

Comroe, Julius H., Jr. *Retro Specro Scope: Insights into Medical Discovery.* Menlo Park, CA: Von Gehr Press, 1978.

Cone, Thomas E., Jr. *History of the Care and Feeding of the Premature Infant.* Boston: Little, Brown, 1985.

———. "L'Hopital Des Enfants-Malades, the World's First Children's Hospital." *Pediatrics* 67, no. 5 (1981): 670.

Crelin, Edmund S. *Functional Anatomy of the Newborn.* New Haven, CT: Yale University Press, 1973.

Desmond, Murdina MacFarquhar. *Newborn Medicine and Society.* Austin, TX: Eakin Press, 1998.

Farr, W. "Mortality of Children in the Principal States of Europe." *Journal of the Royal Statistical Society* 29, no. 1 (1866): 1–12.

Fuchs, Rachel. *Foundlings and Child Welfare in Nineteenth-Century France.* Albany: State University of New York Press, 1984.

———. *Poor and Pregnant in Paris: Strategies for Survival in the Nineteenth Century.* New Brunswick, NJ: Rutgers University Press, 1992.

Gallagher, Mary Barelli. *My Life with Jacqueline Kennedy.* New York: Coronet, 1970.

Garrison, Fielding H. A. B. *History of Medicine.* Philadelphia: W. B. Saunders, 1929.

Jennings, Bojan Hamlin. *Mel: A Biography of Dr. Mary Ellen Avery.* Charleston, SC: Privately published, 2010.

Lincoln, Evelyn. *My Twelve Years with John F. Kennedy.* New York: Bantam Books, 1965.

Meckel, Richard A. *Save the Babies.* Baltimore: The Johns Hopkins University Press, 1990.

Newman, George. *Infant Mortality: A Social Problem.* 1907. Repr. Charleston, SC: Biblilife, 2011.

O'Brien, Michael. *John F. Kennedy: A Biography.* New York: St. Martin's Press, 2005.

O'Donnel, Kenneth P., and Dave Powers, with Joe McCarthy. *"Johnny, We Hardly Knew Ye": Memories of John Fitzgerald Kennedy.* Boston: Little, Brown, 1970.

Parmelee, Arthur Hawley. *Management of the Newborn.* 2nd ed. Chicago: Year Book, 1961.

Patterson, Sandra R., and Lawrence S. Thompson. *Medical Terminology from Greek and Latin.* New York: Whitston, 1996.

Pattle, R. E. "Properties, Function and Origin of the Alveolar Lining Layer." *Nature* 175 (1955): 1125–26.

Philip, Alistair G. S. "The Evolution of Neonatology." *Pediatric Research* 58, no. 4 (2005): 799–815.

———, ed. *Milestones in Neonatal/Perinatal Medicine: Historical Perspectives from NeoReveiws.* Elk Grove, IL: American Academy of Pediatrics, 2010.

Preston, Samuel H., and Michael R. Haines. *Fatal Years: Child Mortality in Late Nineteenth-Century America.* Princeton, NJ: Princeton University Press, 1991.

Rank, Otto. *The Myth of the Birth of the Hero.* New York: Vintage Books, 1960.

Ransel, David L. *Mothers of Misery: Child Abandonment in Russia.* Princeton, NJ: Princeton University Press, 1988.

Rendle-Short, Morwenna, and John Rendle-Short. *The Father of Childcare: Life of William Cadogan (1711–1797).* Bristol: John Wright, 1966.

Rudolph, Arnold J., and Clement Smith. "Idiopathic Respiratory Distress of the Newborn: An International Exploration." *Journal of Pediatrics* 57, no. 6 (1960): 905–21.

Scarpelli, Emile M. *The Surfactant System of the Lung.* Philadelphia: Lea and Febiger, 1968.

Scarpelli, Emile M., Peter A. M. Auld, and Harold S. Goldman. *Pulmonary Disease of the Fetus, Newborn and Child.* Philadelphia: Lea and Febiger, 1978.

Schwartz, Rachel M., Anastasia M. Luby, John W. Scanton, and Russell J. Kellogg. "Effect of Surfactant on Morbidity, Mortality, and Resource Use in Newborn Infants Weighing 500 to 1500 g." *New England Journal of Medicine* 330 (1994): 1476–80.

Silverman, William A. "Incubator-Baby Side Shows." *Pediatrics* 64 (1979): 127.

———. *Retrolental Fibroplasia: A Modern Parable.* New York: Grune and Stratton, 1980.

Smith, Clement A., and Nicholas M. Nelson. *The Physiology of the Newborn Infant.* Springfield, IL: Charles C. Thomas, 1976.

Stevens, Timothy P., and Robert A. Sinkin. "Surfactant Replacement Therapy." *Chest* 131, no. 5 (2007): 1577–82.

Terpstra, Nicholas. *Abandoned Children of the Italian Renaissance: Orphan Care in Florence and Bologna.* Baltimore: Johns Hopkins University Press, 2005.

Thibeault, Donald, and George A. Gregory. *Neonatal Pulmonary Care.* East Norwalk, CT: Appleton-Century-Crofts, 1979.

Thornton, Willis. *The Country Doctor.* New York: Grossett and Dunlap, 1936

Tran, Dinh-DE, and George W. Anderson. "Hyaline-Like Membranes Associated with Disease of the Newborn Lungs: A Review of the Literature." *Obstetrical and Gynecological Survey* 8, no. 1 (1953): 2–3.

Travell, Janet. *Office Hours: Day and Night—The Autobiography of Janet Travell, M.D.* Cleveland, OH: New American Library, 1968.

Weiner, Dora B. *The Citizen Patient in Revolutionary and Imperial Paris.* Baltimore: The Johns Hopkins University Press, 1993.

West, John B. *Respiratory Physiology, People and Ideas.* New York: Published for the American Physiological Society by Oxford University Press, 1996.